DR. DENNIS PERMAN

NEW PATIENTS *EVERY* DAY

How to Build a New Patient Machine and Attract the Right
Number of the Right People Into Your Practice

For permission requests, write to the publisher, addressed Attention: Permissions Coordinator, at the address below.

Dennis Perman, DC
Sexual Wellness Press
129 East Neck Road
Huntington, NY 11743
dennis@sexualwellnesspress.com
www.newpatientseveryday.com

Editing by FirstEditing.com

Layout and Printing by BookBaby.com

Ordering Information: Quantity sales. Special discounts are available on quantity purchases by corporations, associations, and others. For details, contact the Special Sales Department at the address above.

New Patients Every Day/Dr. Dennis Perman—1st ed.

ISBN 978-0-9863977-7-6

TABLE OF CONTENTS

INTRODUCTION

I'm excited to share with you the distilled wisdom of over 35,000 hours of distinctions on how to fill your practice with the highest quality new patients imaginable. I have been coaching chiropractors and wellness professionals for twenty-seven years, and the most common question I get asked is, "How do I get more new patients?" This book offers a series of systems to help every doctor get as many new patients as desired— indeed, new patients every day.

Now, why don't we already get all the new patients we want? The problem is not a lack of new patients. I mean, when you walk down your street, 90% of the people you see are not under chiropractic care, and 99% are not under your care. So, there's certainly no shortage of new patients. There must be something else going on.

My observations, both real-time in the trenches and behind the scenes with thousands of doctors in coaching sessions, have led me to design specific systems that, when implemented properly, should help you develop exactly the practice you want, not only with the number of new patients you prefer, but the kind of new patients that you love to take care of.

Why don't chiropractors already know this? It's because we usually think, if I just had more new patients, that would be the answer. But new patients don't exist in a vacuum. New patients are part of an entire system.

Your practice has dynamics that determine whether or not you can attract new patients, and whether or not you have room to accept and properly serve the new patients you do attract.

Throughout these pages, we're going to be discussing every aspect of generating new patients. What do you have to do in order to get the kind of new patients you especially want? How do you market for them, how do you engage them, how do you get agreement with them so they get the service they need? And what are the characteristic habit patterns of the best new patient getters?

Once you have this material under your belt, you should be able to create exactly the practice you desire—not just the volume and the income, but the kind of patients you love taking care of. As I said, ideal new patients don't exist in a vacuum. Ideal new patients are part of a system.

The purpose of the first chapter of this book is to present the basic fundamental system that determines how likely it is that you will attract new patients, and how ready you are to accept them. Once you understand these foundational concepts, you're ready to learn about the six methods of generating new patients.

The next six chapters each address a major category of new patient attraction strategy: referrals, networking with professionals, public speaking, promotions, Internet marketing, and back-end fronting, which means displaying other valuable health and wellness products and services you recommend so you can reach new people seeking those solutions. Each of these chapters includes not only specific strategies, but also tools and techniques of personal growth and communication that will help you improve your results.

The final chapter puts all the material together to build a new patient machine, to attract as many high-quality new patients as you want.

The end product is that you can attract one or more new patients every day. Or at whatever rate you desire. There's a way to get there, and it's based on the interplay between two natural laws—so to get started in Chapter 1, let's take a look at capacity and attraction—how practices grow.

Dennis Perman, DC, August 2015

CHAPTER 1
Capacity and Attraction—How Practices Grow

I live in a very beautiful home. In fact, right now I'm looking out my window at a picturesque scene—sailboats on a lovely bay, seabirds in the sky, other magnificent houses peeking out through the woods across the water—beautiful.

When I look at the bay, I get this incredible feeling of being connected to something big, being part of nature. But then, I also feel tiny, like a little grain of sand on the beach.

When I look at the bay, I feel empowered. I feel resourceful. But when I turn my attention away from the window, like I just did, for example, and I look at the wall, before too long, those feelings and sensations start to diminish.

In fact, if I look at the blank wall long enough, I may forget the bay is even there. The question is, is the bay still there?

Yes, of course the bay is there. And the moment I turn my attention back to the window and look—*bam!* There are those feelings of connection again. There are those feelings of being large and small, those feelings of being part of nature, something greater.

Our resources, what we have to work with inside of ourselves, are a lot like the bay. When we're focused on our resources, we experience them loud and clear. But if we're not focused on our resources, we may lose touch with them—it may even seem like they're not there, even though they are.

You have inside of you all the resources you could ever need to be able to handle and attract as many new patients as you want. You've been confident somewhere along the line. You've been motivated somewhere along the line. You've been focused and self-disciplined, and confrontational, and authoritative, and positive, and enthusiastic.

All the different qualities you would need in order to be attractive to new patients, you already have.

But the question is, are you focused on those resources when you're in the new patient generating scenario? When you're thinking about how to bring new patients into your practice, get connected to your resources, and you'll put yourself in a position to attract all the new patients that you want.

This brings up an important idea—that, like a glass of water, you have a certain volume. You have a certain amount or capacity you can hold. For example, an 8-ounce glass can hold up to 8 ounces. Now, it could hold 2 ounces. It could hold 4 or 6 ounces. It can hold 7 or 7.99 ounces. But once you get to 8 ounces, the glass can hold no more.

The fact of the matter is, **you can't get 9 ounces into an 8-ounce glass.**

Now, the reason this is so important in the context of building your practice and attracting more new people is that if you're at 8 ounces—in other words, if you're at your capacity—then it doesn't make any sense to try to attract more new people because you simply don't have any room for them.

The first order of business is to make sure you have sufficient capacity to be able to accept the new patients you're looking for.

In fact, this brings up the **first fundamental key to capacity technology:**

There's only two kinds of things in the world—the things you can do something about, and the things you can't do anything about.

And it's the height of insanity to put time, energy, attention, and effort into things you can't do anything about. So, when it comes to generating new patient flow and building the practice you really want, it's critically important that you stay focused on things you can actually do something about.

What somebody else is going to do or not do, you may not have control over, but what you do and don't do, you have a lot of control over. And that's where this process begins.

Most of us have driven a car. You know that when you drive your car, when you put your foot on the gas, you go, and when you put your foot on the brake, you stop.

But what happens when you put your foot on the gas and the brake at the same time? Well, you stop. You might gun the gas against the brake, and you may lurch around a little bit, but you're not going anywhere until you take your foot up off the brake. And when you do, even the gentlest pressure on the accelerator takes you forward.

Which helps us understand the **second fundamental key to capacity technology:**

You can only grow as great as your weaker areas allow.

Now, this is critically important, because you may have been thinking that the weaker area in your practice was not enough new patients, and I'm not even going to say that this isn't the case.

But, until you learn how to develop those aspects of yourself that are weaker in the context of generating new patient flow, then you can't reasonably expect the new patients to flow towards you.

This is how we can take control of our new patient flow. No, you can't control what somebody else does or doesn't do, but you can certainly control your own capacity, and you can certainly control your own attraction.

The New Patients Every Day Systems™ are built on these ideas, so that you get a philosophical foundation for why you're currently at the level of new patients and volume you're currently at, and what kinds of things you're going to need to change in order to move yourself forward.

Capacity Technology™ is one of cornerstones of new patient attraction. You see, you have unlimited potential, but you only have access to some of it, and the portion of your potential that you have access to is called your capacity.

If you want to know your capacity, look around—it's what you've currently got. And as long as you only have access to this amount of your unlimited potential, you can only grow as great as the weaker areas allow.

So, you have to stay focused on the things you can actually do something about in order to grow yourself in those weaker areas, and that will give you access to more of the considerable potential that you, as of yet, have not accessed.

Then, the real question in growing capacity is, where do you have your foot on the brake? Where is the place you're weaker? Where's your capacity limitation? Where are the things that you may need to confront or deal with in order to be able to create the flow of the kind of new patients you're looking for?

That's what we're going to be exploring as we go forward.

Now, there are really two broad categories of capacity limitation.

First, there's **capacity limitation by procedure**, based on what you do, the mechanics or operations of your practice.

To deal with such capacity limitations by procedure, you could choose from six types of procedural improvements or interventions.

You could add hands—in other words, you could get more help. You could add days, or work more hours per day. This gives you more time to be able to process and help more people. You could add speed, one of the most common issues. Moving too slowly or applying your time inefficiently will prevent you from covering all the ground you'd like to cover. So, sometimes you need to just pick up the pace.

Often, there is a capacity limitation in the systems or technology you're using. You may not have a good system for marketing. You may not have a good system for new patient processing. You may need to retool your report of findings. You may not have a good way of educating your patients along the way.

And, your technology may or may not be up to date. So, the key is to be able to understand where your capacity might be limited, and apply one of these fixes.

Now, the sixth one is to add attitude and energy. Even though that seems like it should be on the "be" list, I leave it on the "do" list because everything you do is affected by your attitude and energy.

The second type of capacity limitation occurs at the "be" level, referred to as **capacity limitation by concept and vision**. These elements are dealt with by internal processes. The procedures were dealt with by adding hands or adding days or hours, or systems or speed or technology.

But for the "be" level concepts, the "be" level capacity limitations, you will have to add something internal—affirmations and positive self-talk, for example, or visualizing what you especially want. Setting goals so that you have good targets to aim at, since the mind is target-oriented. Identifying weaker areas and building resources to handle them. In other words, you can reduce or eliminate "be"-level limitations by developing the qualities you would need inside, like more confidence, more motivation, more focus, more discipline, and so on.

You might need to examine your beliefs about new patients. Do you think new patients are scarce when they're really not? Do you think new patients are a burden, or do you look forward to starting new people? Maybe you think you can only handle a certain amount of new patients, when actually you could handle more if you had better systems and a better foundation upon which to process them.

Maybe there's a values conflict; maybe you have mixed emotions, both pleasure and pain stacked up on attracting new patients. Maybe you like the idea of new patients, but you don't like the inconvenience of processing them or the confrontation of getting them to commit to your program of care.

Maybe there are some organizing principles that need to be reorganized. In other words, maybe there are some foundational codes you practice and live by, that either you're not congruently measuring up to, or maybe some of them are outdated or inaccurate and need to be replaced.

You can also deal with capacity limitations by concept and vision with habits of excellence. It may seem like habits are something you do, not something you are, but habits are on the "be" list because they are the sum total of everything you are. They're the manifestation of your being-ness, in reality, how you show up.

This brings up a critical foundational philosophy about being, doing, and having. Being and doing are often considered separately, but they are really part of the same system—the interface between them is attitude and energy on the "do" side, and habits of excellence on the "be" side. When you perform habits of excellence with optimal attitude and energy, you are getting the most out of being and doing, and that generally leads to having, whether it's new patients, money, opportunity, relationships, or whatever.

You see, new patients will only come as part of an overall system of personal and professional growth and development. The system that helps you troubleshoot where your attention is needed is called the Practice Fulfillment Quotient (PFQ). It will show you how to attract and process the ideal number of the ideal kind of new patients.

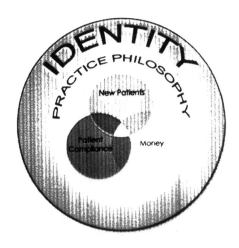

The Practice Fulfillment Quotient (PFQ)

You can see that there are five circles in this model. The three inner circles represent the operations or mechanics of your practice. In essence, they're the "do" steps, though they are also affected by "be"-level conditions. Then we see the two outer circles of this model, representing your identity and your practice philosophy. These are your "be" elements in the Practice Fulfillment Quotient, though of course they are affected by "do"-level actions.

This interplay between being and doing has the three inner circles floating in a matrix of practice philosophy within the ring of identity. So, attracting new patients is obviously both a mechanical operational process, and also a philosophical and vibrational process. The edges of these inner circles are clearly engaging the "be" elements. That's the reason why, even though identity and practice philosophy seem like being, new patients, patient compliance, and money management feel like doing, all five of them require both being and doing. And we're about to dig in to why this is so critical in developing your new patient flow.

I want to point out one more thing to you while we're looking at this particular model. You'll notice that in the center, there's kind of a white triangle with rounded sides.

In fact, this is the graphic representation of your degree of practice fulfillment. Because if you think about it, in order for you to feel fulfilled, all five of these areas need to be in alignment. Your identity has to be a sufficient identity for you to be able to execute what you want to execute at the "be" level. Your practice philosophy, which is the way you express your identity in the context of your practice, needs to be in alignment with both your identity and your mechanics and operations of the practice. Your new patients, while there are certainly specific strategies you need to execute, there is also a sense of self, a sense of identity that goes along with attracting those new patients. You probably know people who don't seem to have to work very hard at it—they just attract lots of new people because their sense of self includes a lot of attraction for new people.

Likewise, the patient compliance circle is going to be at both the "be" and "do" levels because you're going to have to do certain things, but you're also going to have a certain sense of self in order to be able to execute on those things that you need to do.

Likewise, with money and profitability, you will have certain mechanical systems. But you also have some internal vibrational elements that you need to bring into alignment in order for you to be able to have the experience with money that you really desire.

Now, notice that the only place in this model that is completely contained within all five circles is that central white triangle. See, it's inside the identity circle, it's inside the practice philosophy circle, it's inside the new patient circle, it's inside the patient compliance circle, and it's inside the money management circle. Now, we want to be as fulfilled as possible in practice, so how can we make that area larger? We're going to be talking about that throughout the remainder of this chapter. If you look at it, if those inner circles got larger—in other words, the new patient circle, the patient compliance circle, and money management circle got larger—then that would move the sides of the circle, and it would make that internal triangle of fulfillment bigger.

Sometimes the answer isn't necessarily *more*, it's *better*. In other words, you may not need more new patients, you may just need a new patient who is a better fit, who is more suitable for your style of practice, and who you really enjoy engaging and taking care of. So, if that's the case, notice that if these three inner circles move toward the center, then that would also move the sides of the circles, which would enlarge that inner triangle of fulfillment.

So, rather than just attracting more new patients, it's even better to attract more *ideal* new patients. As your new patient compliance and money management gets more ideal, that sets the stage for this inner triangle to get as large as possible, optimizing your sense of fulfillment in practice and in life.

If you like, you can conceptualize that it's like the atlas at the foramen magnum—in alignment, there's a free flow of nerve energy. When your practice fulfillment quotient is wide open, there's a free flow of abundance and satisfaction in your practice.

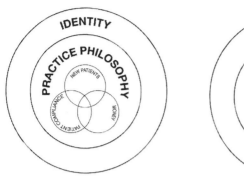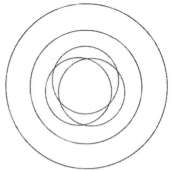

This is the basic philosophy of the PFQ, the Practice Fulfillment Quotient. Let's get more specific about this so we can see precisely how it would influence new patient flow.

It's easy to see that if the new patient circle gets bigger, that inner triangle also gets bigger, increasing practice fulfillment. If it were closer to the center, then that would also make that inner triangle bigger. The trick is to figure out, in the context of this system, what adjustment is required to your new patient strategies and your new patient self-image in order to be able to create more ideal new patients.

We're going to see how to build a new patient machine in Chapter 8, and we're going to get specific about how you can synthesize all the different material from these eight chapters into a new patient system that helps you attract all the new patients you want, New Patients Every Day, and develop the capacity to be able to handle them expediently. But the four big chunks of the new patient machine are for you to target your ideal patient, to build the capacity you need, to set effective goals, and to design a marketing process that generates the new patients you desire.

Five Steps to Target Your Ideal Patient

Your first step at targeting ideal patients is to identify the patients you like—in other words, to distinguish which kinds of people you really love to take care of. Secondly, you need to locate them in their natural habitat; where they're likely to be found. Thirdly, you need to increase your visibility in that location so they notice you and you get their attention. Fourthly, you'll need to learn to close effectively so that you can enroll them, to move the person from being a candidate to actually saying yes, I would like to be your patient.

The fifth step is to make sure that your office procedure and your office plan, your environment, matches up to the kind of people you're looking for. For example, if you want to cater to seniors, then don't expect a lightning-quick office visit because they don't move that quickly at times. Or if you want to have lots of kids coming in, then you wouldn't want to have a lot of low surfaces with small or fragile knick-knacks on them because they're going to get broken or eaten.

These five steps target your ideal patient—identify the kind of person you want, locate them where they're likely to be found, increase your visibility in those locations, learn how to enroll that patient effectively, and then serve those people how they'll be best served. That's how you target your ideal patient.

Once you're doing that, make sure you establish sufficient capacity so you can handle an influx of new patients. You're already aware of the capacity limitations and solutions discussed earlier in this chapter. You can also do a process where you analytically evaluate how much time it takes to see a new patient, to do an office visit, to do a re-exam, and how much time you need each day for other non-patient services like paperwork, meetings, training, returning phone calls, or whatever.

When you take all that data and process it, you can figure out your actual capacity, how many people you can handle. It doesn't make sense for you to set goals unless you know you have (or can develop) capacity to be able to accept and receive them. This is discussed in great detail in Chapter 8.

Next, after targeting ideal patients and developing sufficient capacity, you would need to set appropriate goals, perhaps with a convenient and effective goal-setting system such as the 10%/20% rule.

Introducing the 10%/20% Rule

The 10%/20% rule shows us that a good goal must meet two criteria—it must be believable, and it must be motivating. If the goal is too far away, it may be motivating, but it's not that believable. If it's too close, it may be very believable, but not that motivating. The key is to strike the right balance so it is far enough away to be motivating and close enough to be believable. Typically, the balance between believability and motivation is about 20%. Now, if for you, it's 18% or 24%, no worries; it doesn't matter, the concept is the same. For the purpose of this exercise, we'll use 20%.

It's human nature to want to hit it before we reset it to the next level. There's a problem with this because as you get closer and closer to the goal, it becomes more believable, but less motivating—because you're getting closer to it, so it's getting closer to you. So, as you start to just believe you can do it, but it's not that motivating, this balance is altered, and you typically would decelerate or slow down. This is why sometimes we have trouble hitting our goals because as we get closer and closer to them, we're still aiming at the same goal, and we disturb the proper balance of believability and motivation.

So, the trick is to preserve your momentum and forward thrust by increasing the goal when you get halfway there. This will be discussed in more detail in Chapter 8, but the 10%/20% rule means that you set your goal about 20% from where you are, and then when you get halfway there, about 10% growth, that's when you bump the goal up another 20%, maintaining the balance between believability and motivation.

Now, the final piece of building a new patient machine is to design an effective marketing calendar. And the reason this is so important is because now that you've targeted your ideal patient, now that you know you have sufficient capacity, now that you have goals that you can aim at, now, you have to have a precise strategy for actually connecting all these dots. And the way you do it is by selecting new-patient-generating activities that will attract your ideal patient in the numbers that you're looking for. This will be covered in more detail in Chapters 5 and 8.

Notice, it doesn't have to be only one kind of ideal patient. You may have several kinds of ideal patients. Therefore, you may have several kinds of marketing strategies that you're going to apply. When we talk in more detail about the marketing calendar later on, then you'll have more precision about how to design one. But in essence, Chapters 2-7 supply many different new patient attraction techniques you can feed into your new patient machine once it's built.

Let's spend a little bit of time on the patient compliance circle because, as I said, the new patient flow does not exist in a vacuum, it's part of a system. If you have limitations in any aspect of the system, it could influence your ability to bring in new patients. So, let's talk a little bit about patient compliance.

Patient compliance is your ability to get your patient to commit to a program of care that is in his or her best interest, and also in your best interest as well. Too often doctors absorb the stress of delinquent or uncooperative patients, and it makes us unhappy and eats our capacity. So, getting a patient to comply is more than just attracting nice people, it's training them effectively so that they know what's expected of them, and therefore, that sets the stage for them to have the best experience possible, and also for you to have the best experience possible. Let's explore this in a little more detail.

In order to generate patient compliance, you'll need to develop skills that build your patient visit average, your PVA, the number of visits a patient comes to see you. These skills are referred to as the PVA Skills.

Exploring the Patient Compliance Circle

There are four regions that a patient goes through in their journey in your practice, starting with learning about what you do and how they need to respond, and culminating in a lifetime wellness relationship for you and the patient to enjoy.

We all know that not every patient makes it the entire distance, but the key here is to set the stage for as many people as possible to be able to have the best possible experience. In order to do that, we use the PVA skills to steer them through these four regions of their care.

The first region of care is called basic training. Basic training helps the patients to understand that they're in a different kind of office than they've ever been in before. Often, they've had medical care, and sometimes they've even had some chiropractic care, but they've never been in your office. So, you need to use the first PVA skill to train the patient in the basic behaviors and habits they're going to need to express to get the best possible result in your office. That first PVA skill is your entry procedure. It's the way you bring the patient into your practice, with the centerpiece of it being the ROF, the report of findings.

What goes into a good entry procedure? The front desk CA answers the phone cordially and recognizes the new patient. An appointment is made for a new patient consultation, history, and exam.

Upon arrival at your office, the new patient needs to be greeted effectively by the front desk CA or new patient advocate. Then, the patient has to be directed on how to complete the paperwork, if it hasn't been submitted online already. They submit it, and then they have a seat where the CA guides them, the best seat in the house.

Once they complete the entry paperwork, the CA releases the patient to the doctor for the consultation-history-exam. The doctor does the consultation, history, and exam, then releases the patient back to the CA to schedule the report of findings. The CA makes the appointment and releases the patient. Then, the patient comes back for the report of findings appointment, when the CA receives the patient and makes the release to the doctor for the report of findings.

So you see, there's a procedure that trains the patient to comply, right from the beginning. They learn that yours is an office that works efficiently and on time. Your office sweats the details of excellent service, where patients are guided every step of the way, with the culmination of this being the report of findings.

Now, in my report of findings training, I typically recommend three chunks, three pieces to each report. The first chunk covers the most important questions that are going on in the patient's mind. There are four questions every patient comes in and needs answered in order for them to be able to hear the other things you say. If you don't answer these four questions early on, there is a good chance their minds will be groping around for the answers to these questions and they may not hear the other important stuff that you need them to learn.

These four questions are: Can you help me? What's wrong with me? How long is this going to take? And how much is this going to cost? Then, you need to learn to answer these questions early on in your report of findings. It's not the purpose to go too deeply into this at this time, except to give you the big picture. But it's really important for you to learn how to include the answers to these four questions in the early part of your report of findings.

The second chunk you need to explain is your program of care. You need to make sure your patient knows what your responsibilities are, what their responsibilities are, and how you can keep each other accountable to make sure there is a productive engagement that allows the patient to get the most out of your care, and provides you with the least stressful and most enjoyable experience in taking care of that patient.

Once you've answered the patient's four questions, once you've explained your program of care to them, then it's critically important that you finish your report of findings with a commitment. The commitment portion of the report of findings is perhaps the most important part.

At the end of your report, you must say to your patient, "Well, Mr. Patient, I've answered all your questions, and I've explained the program of care. You know what your responsibilities are, and what my responsibilities are. Now, we're approaching the moment of truth. I can't want this more than you do. You have to be committed to this program of care. This may not be easy, but it's essential for you to do what I've explained to get the results you want. Can I count on you to follow through on this program of care exactly the way I've outlined it to you?"

And you extend your hand, palm up, and you get an eye gaze and a smile. Don't say anything more. Get a handshake—that's a verbal contract, because the key is for the patient to understand that you're talking about them. You're not just talking in general terms about somebody. You're talking about *them* and their body, and this is what they need. They must understand that they've got to commit to the program of care. And they will never commit to it unless you exact that commitment, unless you cause them to get into agreement with you about the follow-through on this program of care. That's the basic training section.

The second region that a patient goes through is what I call "communicating the message." Once they have your basic training, now you get the chance to put your spin on chiropractic. One of the most glorious things about being a chiropractor is that, given the basic fundamental philosophy, you can come at chiropractic care from a variety of different angles, different techniques, different political orientations, and different sub-specialties. So, you get to communicate your message to the patient, and the PVA skill that you used to do that is your patient education process.

There are any number of ways for you to do this. You can do health care classes. You can do advanced health care talks. You can do wellness orientation workshops. You can put posters up on your wall and direct people's attention toward them. You can use patient literature. But the most powerful way to communicate the message of chiropractic is through one-on-one patient education done in little bites, little tidbits on every visit. This way, you put another brick in the wall every single time the patient comes in, and you help them understand what they need to know to not only follow through on their commitment, but to understand what chiropractic is so that they can have it in their life forever, and so they can also recommend that others have the opportunity to do so.

This takes us to the third region of patient care, which I call "case management beyond relief." In other words, there will come a time when your patient is feeling better. The way that they've probably been trained before their time with you is that once they're feeling better, they don't need to go to the doctor anymore. They tell the doctor where it hurts. They only go to the doctor while they're sick.

That's not true in a chiropractic office because we work on causes, not only on the patient's symptoms. The tool that we use in order to guide the patient through case management beyond relief is the re-exam or re-examination mini report, also known as a progress report.

In that report, you want to help the patient understand why they need care beyond the point where they're feeling better. It's new to them. They don't understand. So, you may want to use some kind of technology, a NeuroInfiniti or an Insight to show them where they are in their nerve system health, whether they're feeling symptoms or not. You can also do it with ranges of motion or finding taut and tender fibers—but it's really important that you demonstrate a need for continued nerve system and brain care beyond the point they're feeling better.

You can also use a simple metaphor here, the fire alarm. You can say, "Well, Mr. Patient, if you heard a fire alarm ringing, then you'd assume there was a fire somewhere. And if all you did was shut off the fire alarm, then you would be in jeopardy because the fire would still be burning. This is a lot like your symptoms and the underlying problem. The pain you have seems like the problem, but it's not the problem. It tells you, you have a problem. And if all we do is shut off the pain, without fixing the underlying cause, that's like shutting off the fire alarm without putting out the fire."

Easy metaphors like these make it a little bit more accessible for the patient to be able to understand, because it's a huge paradigm shift for them as to why they need care beyond the point where they feel better. But it's critical for their ultimate well-being for you to be able to convey this to them.

That takes us to the fourth region of patient care, which I call the "lifetime patient." A lifetime patient is not somebody who comes in once a week for life, even though they may choose to do so. A lifetime patient is somebody who understands the value of chiropractic care and who chooses to have it as part of their life going forward.

The PVA skill that I use to convert on this fourth region is your recall system. Again, it's not the purpose of this chapter to go into every detail of the recall system, but it is critical for you to have a recall system, both to be able to recall people if they miss a visit, but also, when somebody leaves or fades, for you to be able to contact them and re-engage them as a patient, based on their needs, as you go forward.

These four PVA skills can be found between pages 215 and 230 in the book *The Masters Guide for the 21st Century Chiropractor*, and they can also be found on the *Mastering The Message* album, available at the Masters Circle Store. (For more information see the Resources page following Acknowledgments.)

Exploring the Money Management Circle

Let's move on to the money management circle. The money circle is also an important part of new patient acquisition and attraction because if you have issues about money at the "be" level, then that will restrict or hinder your ability to attract new people. And if you have strategic or mechanical issues with money—poor collections or poor money management—or issues with getting your own bills paid, then you'll be consumed with those kinds of stresses. That will eat resources and energy that make it less likely that you can attract the number of new patients you desire. So, understanding the money management circle is essential.

Again, it's not our purpose to address this completely here, but there are a couple of important points to be made. At the "be" level, the money management circle is affected by prosperity consciousness. In other words, it's critical for you to have an abundance mentality. It's not about hoarding, it's about accumulation, because if you manage your money effectively, especially if you're willing to create a financial master plan, then that gives you a specific series of strategies by which you can become wealthy. And by being wealthy, that allows you to participate in all the "be" elements of prosperity consciousness, which will help you attract more new people because you won't look at a new patient like a hungry man looks at a T-bone steak. You'll have a sense of benevolence, a sense of love, a sense of service orientation that will guide your attraction rather than need and lack.

You can find a model of the financial master plan on page 141 of *The Masters Guide*, but simply, it's just six numbers you would calculate and use to figure out your ultimate financial needs and wants. What's your average monthly office overhead? What's your average monthly home expenses? What's your average monthly income tax? Add those three numbers together, and that's your basic nut, or your fixed monthly overhead; in essence, your break-even point.

Most doctors who are not spilling or raiding their reserves in order to be able to pay their bills are functioning at least at this break-even point. But there are three other aspects of the financial master plan: to design a savings plan so that you become wealthy, to reduce your debt to zero in a reasonable amount of time, and to create a fun budget so that you entertain yourself in a manner to which you'd like to become accustomed. (If this is substantially more than your break-even point, remember to figure in your additional income tax.)

When you put these six numbers together, they create a target for you, a financial master plan to target monthly income, from which you can figure out how many office visits and new patients you need in order to be able to get to that target.

Now, at the "do" level, you use business acumen to develop your financial policies and procedures. You charge a certain fee for your services based on your policy, and collect that the best you can. The amount you collect per visit is called your Office Visit Average, or OVA.

If you take your financial master plan target monthly income and divide it by your OVA, you'll see how many office visits you'll need. And if you divide this number of office visits by your PVA, you'll see how many new patients you would need to generate that target income.

How the Three Inner Circles Fit Together

So, this is how these three mechanical circles fit together. If your financial master plan is $30,000 a month, and your OVA is $50, then $30,000 divided by $50 is 600 office visits, so you'd need 600 visits to hit your financial master plan target income.

If you have a 30 PVA, meaning your average patient comes in 30 times, then that means that to get to 600 office visits, you need 20 new patients; 600 office visits divided by 30 visits per patient. Notice, if your average patient comes in 40 times, you only need 15 new patients to get to 600 office visits. If your average patient comes in 50 times, then you only need 12 to get to 600 office visits. Also, notice that to get to 30,000, if your OVA is actually $75 instead of $50, then you'd only need 400 office visits instead of 600. But notice that if your OVA is $30 instead of $50, then to get to 30,000, you'd need to be at 1,000 office visits.

Understanding how these numbers fit together will pave the way for unlimited new patients for you. These distinctions are lurking below the surface for most of us, without us fully grasping the significance of them and understanding how they work together. That's why we're discussing this up front, because you can't get to the new patient flow you're looking for unless you see how new patients fit into this system.

Your collections ratio is the amount of money you earn that you actually collect. Theoretically, it should be 100%, but in most practices it's not, because there are third-party payers that have to be dealt with. There are patients who may not pay you completely. There are hardship situations where you may opt to accept less money. So, it's important for you to recognize that your collections ratio will determine what portion of your services rendered you actually get in your hand.

Your case average is the amount of money you make per case. If you take the example we used before, that your OVA, the amount of money you collect per visit is $50 and your PVA, the amount of visits that a patient comes in is 30, then your case average is 30 visits times $50, or $1,500.

Why is that important? If your goal is to get to $30,000/month and you make $1,500 a case, then you need 20 cases each month. This helps you understand the number of new patients you need to get to your goals. (These ideas are discussed more fully in *The Edge of Prosperity* album— see Resources.)

Exploring the Identity Circle

We've spent a lot of time talking about the "do" elements. Now, let's talk a little bit about "being." Your identity is who you are. Your identity is your sense of self. It's your self-image, your self-concept.

Why is this important in the context of new patients? If you believe yourself to be a great new patient getter, then not only will you likely get more new patients, but all the different actions, steps, and strategies that you need to do will come more easily to you because your belief is that it's simply who you are. In fact, we often say at The Masters Circle that who you are determines how well what you do works.

And this is a critical distinction that helps you recognize why those "be" elements are so vital in the context of new patient acquisition. (If you want to know more about this particular idea, you can listen to the album called *The Identity of a Healer*.)

Exploring the Practice Philosophy Circle

Your practice philosophy is your identity in the context of the practice. In other words, your practice philosophy is who you are as a chiropractor. There are many different shades of difference and gradients here, but there are three basic categories.

There are musculoskeletal chiropractors, who focus on patients' conditions and providing relief. There are traditional chiropractors, who are subluxation based and focus on finding and correcting nerve interference. And there are wellness chiropractors, interested in helping the patient develop lifestyle habits that are consistent with a better quality of life and greater longevity.

None of these are necessarily more correct or incorrect than the others. In fact, all are absolutely necessary. Most of us create a personalized blend of these three practice philosophies. What's your personal blend? (If you want to find out more about this particular idea, check out the *Tools of Mastery* album.)

Why the PFQ is Important in the New Patient Attraction Process

Why did we spend so much time on the Practice Fulfillment Quotient in a book on new patients?

In order for you to be able to attract new patients, you have to have sufficient capacity to receive them, and the PFQ is your optimal tool for troubleshooting capacity limitations.

You can't get 9 ounces into an 8-ounce glass, so this discussion helps you decide where to put your energy to grow in your weaker areas, and improve both the size and the orientation of the inner circles, which then grows the fulfillment area at the center. Remember the metaphor of the foramen magnum—you don't want this area of fulfillment closed down. You want it open wide so that abundance can flow in your direction.

Now you can see how this actually works, and why I made the point before about the capacity limitations by procedure at the do level and by concept and vision at the be level, and why we need to be aware of the interface between being and doing, attitude and energy on the do list, and habits of excellence on the be list.

Riding the Interface Between Being And Doing

We need both being and doing to have what we want. No one can create what they want with pure being or pure doing—even if it sounds possible theoretically, it's not likely in reality. We have to find the right blend of being and doing for our particular desired outcomes.

To remind you, you solve do-level limitations by adding hands, days, hours, speed, systems or technology, or adding attitude and energy, which I call the interface between being and doing on the do side. You address limitations at the be level with affirmation, visualization, goal setting, resource building, beliefs, values, organizing principles or habits of excellence, which I call the interface between being and doing from the be side.

The way to have what you want is to ride the interface between being and doing, which means that you perform habits of excellence with optimal attitude and energy.

Eliminate your capacity limitations with be and do solutions and fixes. Then, work on riding the interface between being and doing by practicing habits of excellence with optimal attitude and energy, and see what happens to your new patient flow. You'll find yourself attracting New

Patients Every Day, or at whatever rate you choose, based on the capacity and attraction you develop.

This may seem to be a rather philosophical beginning to what will ultimately be an extremely practical book, but it's essential that you understand that new patients don't exist in a vacuum. New patients manifest as a result of satisfying the various parts of this system. If new patients are not flowing, there's interference in this system, and if they are, there isn't. The logic is unmistakable.

As we go forward, the next six chapters will give you specific strategies. You'll learn how to get referrals, how to network with professionals, how to use public speaking effectively, how to do effective promotions, how to use social media productively, how to use your specialized products and services to attract new patients with what I call "back-end fronting," and ultimately, in Chapter 8, you'll discover how to build the new patient machine of your dreams that will create the practice that you really want.

Points to Remember

1. The two dynamics of growth are capacity, how much you can hold, and attraction, the power to fill that capacity.

2. You can't get 9 ounces into an 8-ounce glass.

3. There are two kinds of things—things you can do something about, and things you can't. Focus on things you can do something about.

4. You can only grow as great as your weaker areas permit. Build resources to handle weaker areas.

5. There are five areas of practice fulfillment—identity, practice philosophy, new patients, patient compliance, and money management.

6. Capacity can be limited at the be or do level, and there are specific tools you can use to handle them. Use the PFQ to troubleshoot your capacity limitations.

Actions to Take

1. Calibrate where you are in each of the five areas of the PFQ by rating yourself 1-5, with 1 meaning you are not very accomplished in that area, and 5 meaning you are very accomplished in that area. Write down your findings, to be compared later as you incorporate the ideas in this book.

2. Create a baseline of your current new patient flow—write down how many patients you have attracted on average over the last six months, last year, or the last two years.

Questions to Ponder

1. Do you think you have more of a challenge with capacity or attraction?

2. Why do you think you attract patients at your current rate? Are you taking enough action? Do you have sufficient vision?

3. Where are some of your capacity limitations, and what could you begin to do today to address one of them?

This foundation is designed to show you the basic elements of new patient attraction, and how to build the capacity to accept and receive the new patients you attract. In Chapter 2, we'll dig into referrals, and you'll get some specific, practical tools so you can start bringing in new patients every day.

CHAPTER 2

Referrals Made Easy

In Chapter 1, we talked about the fundamental philosophy of New Patients Every Day, the interplay between building capacity and filling it with attraction. First you build capacity, then you fill it with attraction, then you build more capacity and fill that with attraction. You build capacity by reducing or eliminating the interference in the flow of abundance. You have unlimited potential, and there is more than enough success and victory to go around, especially since everyone defines it somewhat differently.

But there is a common denominator between all of the methods of building a great practice—you have to be able to recruit the clientele you love to serve, and learn to serve them so they comply with your recommendations, whatever you believe is in the patient's best interest.

No matter how you define your target—in new patients, office visits, money, or however you choose to measure it, there is a formula that will get you there, some combination of new patients, visits per patient, and dollars per visit. Your target income has to be based on these three numbers. While this book is focused on increasing the number of new patients, you have to be conscious of the systems you apply and what each new patient yields as a contribution toward your target. You'll do better faster when you focus on finding and engaging the kinds of new patients that would be ideal for your formula for chiropractic success.

For example, let's say you want to collect $30,000 per month, and you collect $50 per visit. That means you would need to see 600 office visits a month or about 150 a week, to collect $30,000.

$$\$30,000 = 600 \text{ OVs} \times \$50$$

You could get to 600 office visits by seeing 20 new patients a month thirty times each, or 30 new patients twenty times each, or fifteen new patients forty times each, or twelve new patients fifty times each—these are all formulas to get you to 600 office visits.

$$600 \text{ OVs} = 30 \text{ NPs} \times 20 \text{ PVA}$$
$$600 \text{ OVs} = 20 \text{ NPs} \times 30 \text{ PVA}$$
$$600 \text{ OVs} = 15 \text{ NPs} \times 40 \text{ PVA}$$
$$600 \text{ OVs} = 12 \text{ NPs} \times 50 \text{ PVA}$$

The question is, which kind of new patient do you prefer?

Depending on your practice philosophy and your patient compliance, you will have a higher or lower PVA, and that will require a proportionately lower or higher number of new patients.

Therefore, your best new patient strategy is based on attracting those patients who are a good fit with your practice model, so they and you have the best experience possible, and you reclaim capacity that would been taken up with people who really aren't a good fit for you.

Long-Handled Spoons and the Meaning of Life

Once there was a seeker who wanted to know the meaning of life, and he heard there was an oracle who could help him. He went to visit the oracle high on a mountaintop, and said, "Oh great Oracle, please tell me the meaning of life!"

The oracle waved his arm... there was a puff of smoke... and they found themselves in a dark cave. In the middle of the cave was a large cauldron of brown, bubbling fluid. Sitting around the cauldron were men and women, emaciated, starving, unable to eat the soup because all they had were these long-handled spoons, and they couldn't figure out a way to maneuver the spoon to scoop up the soup and put it in their mouths.

"This is Hell," said the oracle.

He waved his arm again, and again there was a puff of smoke... and they found themselves in a dark cave. In the middle of the cave was a large cauldron of brown, bubbling fluid. Sitting around the cauldron were men and women, but these men and women were smiling, happy, and well-fed. You see, they had learned to use the long-handled spoons to feed their friends across the cauldron, and be fed themselves the same way.

"This is Heaven," said the oracle. And that was really all the seeker needed to know.

When I was in practice, if a patient came to me I felt could be served better by one of my local chiropractic colleagues, I sent them over there. My feeling was that there were many new patients out there, and if I filled my capacity with those who weren't as good a fit, I wouldn't have as much room for those who were more ideal. Plus, I wanted the patient to get the best service possible, and if I felt the patient would do better with another doctor of chiropractic, I referred them out.

It all stems from an underlying belief that there are more than enough new patients. Like I said in Chapter 1, if you walk down your street, 90% of the people you see are not under chiropractic care, and 99% are not under your care. As we begin our new patient strategies for this chapter, keep in mind that you want to concentrate on attracting the kinds of patients you love to serve, as many as possible.

Attracting Referrals

Let's start talking about new patient strategy.

The most general of all the techniques of attracting new patients is referral. Often this is an encounter between you and someone you know or meet, though there's a whole area of referral revolving around professional relationships, which we're going to leave for Chapter 3.

Now, we're going to concentrate on the fundamental principles of the referral process, and provide examples of one-on-one conversations to show you how you can pick up on cues people give you to know the best way to attract them toward being your patient.

The Structure of the Referral Process

The basic format of any referral encounter has three parts, but before you can engage in the new patient scenarios, there are two preconditions to be aware of, and two skills you'll want to develop. First, you must be able to envision what you would like to happen in the referral encounter, no matter what the scenario. Begin with the end in mind, we learned from Stephen Covey. So to generate outcome clarity, think about what you want to occur based on your interaction with this person, and visualize a successful result—it will help you gravitate toward behaviors that work toward that outcome.

Secondly, you must gain rapport with the person you are about to engage. Rapport means an atmosphere of comfort, of liking, a bond or connection that paves the way for good communication and an honest exchange between you.

We tend to think that liking someone is an emotional event, but oddly, it isn't—it's a neuro-mechanical event. Let's look at this term and see what it means.

The way you perceive your environment, including everyone and everything in it, is dependent on your ability to interpret the input your brain and nerve system pick up—your senses give you a conduit to experience the world around you, including your sight, hearing, touch, taste, and smell. These body functions stem from your nerve system—the word *neuro* relates to the nerve system.

The word *mechanical*, of course, means machine-like, automatic, unconscious, reflex, or involuntary. So the word *neuro-mechanical* means that your nerve system picks up certain input and has a typical, usual pattern of responses to it.

That suggests that liking someone, or feeling connected to them, is based on reflex responses that come from the way your nerve system picks up and interprets what's going on. That's the reason you can meet someone at a party and instantly feel *I like this person* or *I don't like this person*, though you may have little fact or detail to validate those impressions. It's an automatic feedback system, and in most people who are unaware of this, an uncontrollable compulsion to feel good or not feel good around certain people.

The good news is, once you are aware of this tendency, you can choose or refine both the way you show up and the way you perceive those around you. You can learn to produce pleasing or connected experiences with people because you are noticing what makes them like they are, and how you can create a good feeling between you and them, based on a simple principle:

> People who are like each other tend to like each other,
> and
> people who are not like each other tend to not like each other.
> −Anthony Robbins

The first secret to creating the kind of connection that leads to developing a quality relationship is the ability to cause someone to see you as like them, so they tend to like you. If they see you as not like them, they will tend to not like you.

How can we willfully start this process of liking in motion?

Remember, the input your nerve system is seeking is sensory in nature, so the first key is to become sensitive to the way the other person is showing up; in other words, their tendencies and patterns—facial expressions, posture, movements, voice qualities like tempo or volume, word choice—those perceptible details that we mostly overlook, yet which hold a treasure trove of distinctions that allow us to enter the other person's world with respect.

Rapport begins when we are willing to detect the subtle signs that make someone uniquely them, so we can honor those patterns instead of ignoring them like almost everyone else does. This simple observation sets the stage for you to respond in a respectful, healthy, inviting way by doing something that may seem counterintuitive, but once you understand it, makes a lot of sense.

The key is, you want to give the person back his or her own patterns, by matching and mirroring—in other words, picking up their facial expression, posture, voice qualities, and other characteristics—and reflect those back to the other person. In this way, you are "like them," which makes them tend to "like you." This initiates a feeling of comfort, connection, and liking.

It sounds too simple, too good to be true, but try this simple exercise with someone—you won't even have to explain it, just try it.

Have a conversation with someone as you usually would, but see if you can notice how quickly or slowly they tend to talk. Deliberately speak at the same rate they do—it will take a few attempts to get good at this, but everyone has the natural ability to do this, and you do, too. Notice what happens when you speak at the same rate they do—they will tend to smile, lean in slightly toward you, relax, most of what you might expect when someone likes you.

Now, vary the tempo of your talking, to make it faster or slower, and see what happens—they will tend to seem less connected to you, may lean away slightly, or lose their smile and sense of comfort. Then, shift back to their usual speed, and see them return to the more comfortable demeanor.

This may take a little practice, but within a few trials you will convince yourself that gaining rapport has nothing to do with someone's character, but rather is based on the neuro-mechanical patterns that either fit or don't fit—and a skillful and dedicated communicator can observe patterns that will feel good, and reproduce them willfully.

Match or mirror posture, facial expression, tempo of movement or speech, word choice, and breathing, and you can generate a deep connection with someone, at will, any time you choose, even someone you do not yet know or with whom you have no previous relationship.

As you become more adept at this easily learned skill, you will find that breathing patterns—rate, depth, location in the chest, and other subtleties—are among the most profound ways to connect with someone.

The Three Parts of the Referral Encounter

Once you know your outcome and are able to gain and maintain rapport, we can explore the referral encounter, which is composed of three chunks—first, you must ask targeting questions that focus the conversation on your desired result to get this person to begin as a patient, or to refer someone who then begins as a patient.

Examples of such targeting questions would be, "Say, you're married, aren't you?" or, "You've got a couple of kids, don't you?" or, "You play racquetball with three buddies, right?"

Notice, that these questions are all statements turned into questions by a tag line, also known as a tie-down. Making a statement and finishing with a little question makes the statement into a question, and this is very handy in the targeting section.

You can also target the individual before you if he or she is not already a patient—the language is very similar. For example, "Say, I've seen you around this health club several times. You seem interested in being as healthy and fit as possible, aren't you?" or, "I couldn't help noticing you moving your neck around, like it's bothering you, am I guessing right?"

Whether you are aiming at the target before you or encouraging a referral, once you have agreement on the targeting questions, you move into the second part of the referral encounter, the leverage phase.

Some people misinterpret leverage to mean coercion, force, or arm-twisting, and that is not the intention at all. Leverage means using the person's values to move them toward a decision or conclusion that serves their best interests. If your intention is to get one over on or take advantage of someone, I wish you wouldn't use these tools, as they are too powerful to fall into the wrong hands.

You know, if you go to the hardware store a buy a hammer, you can build a house or bash in someone's skull; it's the same hammer, it's just how you use it. If you ethically engage someone to improve the quality of their lives, you have no ulterior motives and it's completely appropriate that the experience will prove fruitful for you both.

Gain leverage by asking questions that elicit values based on the target you established in the first part. If you asked about someone's spouse and they replied that they did indeed have one, your target is specified, and you could continue, "I ask because most of our patients and practice members want their spouses to get a checkup once they realize how great it is to be under chiropractic care, like you do. Tell me, do you think it's a good idea for your spouse to get a checkup?"

Or, if you are aiming for a friend your patient mentioned was suffering from a health problem, you could ask, "You know how we do things around here—do you think your friend is a good candidate to respond to our approach?"

Leverage questions are designed to uncover a value—health, support, love, a mutual interest or hobby, or shared commitments and responsibilities, for example.

If you have targeted effectively, and elicited a significant enough value, the final chunk of the referral encounter flows right out of the second one—the closing. Closing questions are intended to bring the encounter to conclusion by calling for a decision.

For example, if you are following the spousal referral strategy, and you have a clear target and sufficient leverage, you would then ask, "So, it seems that you would prefer that your wife come in for a checkup—what do you think is the best way to set that up? Would you like to bring her with you next visit, or would you two rather come to our health care class on Tuesday evening at seven thirty?"

Notice that I offer a choice between yes and yes—this is called a double bind (Zig Ziglar called it an alternative choice close) because it offers two options, both of which lead to your desired outcome. Note that ethically, the choices must also suit the best interests of the patient or prospect.

Four-Part Closing

To set up your closing questions, you may want to apply a closing format I call "four-part closing."

The first part of a four-part closing is to summarize the key points you learned about the person's current level of health and wellness, and any key points you made that were perceived to be relevant.

The second and third parts of four-part closing are your motivational parts, moving the person toward the benefits of saying yes and away from the consequences of saying no. This is your interpretation of the data you collected that you restated when you summarized in the first part of the closing. Here's where you show how the person is better off with you than without you.

Finally, the fourth part of your closing is the closing question.

So let's see what this might sound like in a few typical scenarios. First, we're going to look at a conversation in your office with a current patient that demonstrates a good method of asking for a referral. Then, you'll get an example of meeting someone outside your office and encouraging them to come in to begin care.

With an Active Patient

Let's look at an exchange that could happen in any office. Let's say you have a patient who is a married woman, under care for a few weeks and getting good results. The outcome you want is to persuade her to refer her husband. You have completed her adjustment for today, and you have effectively matched and mirrored her, so you have a solid rapport.

You say something like, "We did good work here today, Mary, you seem to be coming along beautifully. Before you head home, may I ask you a few questions?"

She will say yes, and you continue, "You're married, aren't you?" This is your targeting question. When she confirms her marital status, move into your leverage questions.

"So many of our patients bring in their spouses for a checkup, and I noticed that your husband has not been in for an exam. Does he go to another chiropractor?"

If yes, congratulate her on her husband taking responsibility to stay well, and if no, continue your questioning.

"Do you think it's important to have someone taking care of his brain, nerve system, and spinal health care needs?" Usually this will elicit a yes response, and now you have some leverage, her value on having him be healthy. If you think you need more leverage, you can drive it home by saying, "You've seen it yourself how chiropractic care helps in so many ways; do you think he'd benefit from coming in for a checkup?" Again, this usually gets a yes, and you can move into your closing.

"So let me get this right—no one's taking care of your husband's brain, spine, and nerve system, and you think he could benefit from a checkup, at least to find out his current health status and confirm that he's fine, or pick up on any problems early enough to avoid unnecessary suffering. Do I have that right?"

She'll say yes, and you can finish up with, "So, what do you think we ought to do about that? Would you like to bring him with you next time you come in, or would you two prefer to come to our health care class next Tuesday so he can decide for himself?"

At the Health Club

How about if you're at the health club, and you see someone there who seems to fit the description of your ideal patient. You wait for an opportune moment, then you match and mirror to gain rapport. If you're on the treadmill next to someone, this is easy; just match your pace to his or hers and there will be a quick connection formed.

This person is the target, but you still have to find out if he or she is a candidate for your care, so begin probing with leverage questions to elicit values.

"Say, I haven't seen you at the club before, did you just join? I could tell from your workout that you are in good shape. I guess health and fitness are important to you, huh? What do you do to keep your brain and nerve system in shape? Oh, I'm not surprised, most people don't know too much about the brain and nerve system, but actually, it's important in health and fitness—in fact, all your body functions depend on your brain and nerve system. Does that seem like something you'd like to know more about, to improve your workout and get more out of your fitness training? Well, I thought you might be interested—I'm Dr. Perman, I help people like you all the time, that's why I brought it up. Which would work better for you—would you like to come to my free class Tuesday at seven thirty, or would you prefer to just come in to my office for a complimentary consultation?"

Opportunities for dialogues like this abound, so pay attention, watch and listen for openings to have such conversations with people and get some experience, for their good and also yours.

The Three-A-Day Game

One of the simplest and most powerful ways to attract referrals is to play the three-a-day game. To play, choose three people from your appointment book each day, mark their travel card or record with a yellow sticky note labeled "3/day" and you're ready to play. Those people become your three-a-day players, and the game is to get them to refer someone. Pick people you believe know someone who would be a great patient, and while you may talk chiropractic all day to all of your patients, you only close these three times.

At first, you may think, only three times each day? That's not very much. Yet, if you ask for referrals three times each day, five office days per week and four weeks per month, that's fifteen attempts each week and sixty per month. What do you expect your closing ratio to be? If you close ten percent, that would be six new patients each month. Get to twenty per cent, and that's twelve new patients per month. Could you imagine refining your skill so you could close a third? That would be twenty new patients each month.

Also, keep in mind, you're not asking strangers—these are warm leads, people who know you, like you, and like chiropractic—because those are the ones you pick from your appointment book.

This is a consistency game—you must play every day to make it work. Also, don't mistakenly think that if three-a-day is good, five-a-day is better. You're better off with fewer trials and more focus. Remember, the sunshine may warm the countryside, but focus the rays through a magnifying glass, and it can start a fire! You want your energy focused like that, on just three people each day, at least when you're first learning the game.

When you get good at this, and your batting average is solid, you can expand the game to play outside your office—it takes more skill, but it's very exciting. You can play one, two, or three-a-day inside your office, and one, two, or three-a-day outside your office—just play the same number each day, and keep track of your results—for planning purposes, and also to reflect on your impact on your community.

For example, if you play three-a-day inside and get fifteen new patients out of sixty trials, that would be a 25% closing ratio. If your goal is fifteen new patients, then that's all you need to do! If your goal is thirty, then you need to plan other activities to bring in the other fifteen.

Or, you can become more skillful and improve your batting average. However you choose to play, this is one of the most productive new patient attraction techniques known.

Now let's look at some of the finer points of technique in generating referrals.

The Four Filters of Connection

If you want to connect with someone elegantly, observe their communication style and use communication that works for them. Here are four ways to interpret who you're dealing with, called the four filters of connection—representational system, basic personality style, metaprogram formation, and advanced personality typing.

Filter 1: Representational System

Let's talk about the first filter of connection: representational system.

Representational system refers to the part of the individual's brain that is used most dominantly. Visual people use the seeing part of their brain, Auditory people use the hearing part of their brain, and Kinesthetic people depend more on the feeling part of their brain. You can easily tell these types apart by monitoring their pace of speech, movement, and breathing.

Visuals move and speak quickly, because they have pictures flashing through their minds and are trying desperately to keep up with them, because one picture is worth a thousand words. They'll stand with a more erect posture (trying to see), breathe high in their chests, and use words like *see, look, viewpoint, or picture*. Their eyes tend to focus from the midline upward, as if they are surveying the horizon.

Auditories are more moderately paced and toned, because they're paying attention to the way things sound. They'll have more melodious voices, breathe in the midline of their chests, stand a bit more relaxed, and tend to choose words like *hear, ask, call, or sound*. Their eyes tend to remain in and around the midline, as if they are following what they hear to decide where to look.

Kinesthetics speak and move slower, with their breathing low in their abdomen and often hardly speak, preferring to communicate with touching and emotion. They'll choose words like *handle, grasp, solid, or warm*. Their eyes tend to remain midline and down, seeking their feelings, emotions, and sensations.

When you've determined whether someone is visual, auditory, or kinesthetic, address them with a similar pace—talk fast to visuals, moderately to auditories, and slowly to kinesthetics.

Match and mirror their posture, movements, facial expressions, and tonalities, and you'll create a deep rapport that sets the stage for better overall communication. Once you have rapport, you can go to the next screen, personality style.

Filter 2: Personality Style

Now that you have a sense of the part of the brain the person tends to access primarily, we can look at the second filter of connection: basic personality style.

People tend to fall into one of four categories, or some blend of these four—driver, expressive, analytical, and amiable. There are many off-shoots of this typing system—DISC model, birds, dogs, and other colorful interpretations. I prefer these descriptions because for me they most clearly exemplify the key characteristics of each style.

Let's talk about **drivers**.

Drivers are decisive action takers who are task-oriented and know what they want—results. They are problem solvers who tend to assume the leader's role. They can be indifferent or aloof, and get bored with repetitive work. They are self-starting and determined, and are usually fast-paced change-makers. They can usually be identified by their directness and certainty.

Drivers don't like small talk, so cut to the chase when communicating with them, especially in the context of asking for referrals. They respond to a direct approach, so just come at them and propose the referral, and then let them take the lead—if it's a right fit for them, they will close themselves on it, and if not, there isn't much you can do to change that.

Now let's discuss **expressives**.

Expressives are friendly, colorful, and enthusiastic, and love connecting with people. They are optimistic, fun-loving, and often loudly and passionately express their viewpoints in conversation. They are also fast-paced, but tend to be less definite than drivers, staying flexible and gregarious, where drivers might prefer to be more isolated by nature. They usually like touching, feeling, and hugging, and have magnetic personalities to attract others to their causes. This makes them good at helping you recruit candidates for care.

They love ideas and creativity, and are both motivated and motivating, making them effective at generating interest in your office if they dial into helping you bring in more people. Their engaging personalities translate well to encouraging people in any context, so inserting your office into that algorithm can be very productive.

Expressives are usually big picture people rather than detail-oriented, so don't expect them to be able to carry a complicated message for you—keep it simple and uplifting, and they can fill your office with their family members, coworkers, neighbors, and friends.

Let's examine the **analyticals**.

Analyticals thrive on fact, detail, and accuracy. They love data and information, and will respond to scientific validation as well as a skillfully developed argument. They are calculating, straightforward, and questioning, and are slower-paced in spite of being hard workers, because it takes time to consider the assortment of intellectual perspectives available to them, though they tend to be task-oriented like drivers in getting their objectives met.

Their precision makes them follow the rules and keeps their standards high. They are often dry and clinical, as they are focused primarily on the content of your communication rather than the style. You'll have to earn their trust by being correct in your explanations to them, as they will frequently test your input by researching it themselves. They want to know your policies so they can adhere to them, and respond badly to sloppiness, inexact behaviors, and waffling. Give them "just the facts" and they keep their balance and know how to react.

In the referral scenario, analyticals can handle more detail about the brain and nerve system than drivers or expressives. These are the patients you can make a scientific proof to, and when they grasp it they can become skillful at referring, especially other analyticals who speak their language.

Finally, let's consider **amiables**.

Amiables are consistent, pleasant, polite, and warm. They are kind, relationship-driven, and family-oriented, and prefer the status quo. They are also rules-followers like analyticals, but more because they prefer not to confront change than to adhere to a detailed fact sheet. They tend to be slower-paced and less decisive, but they are good workers at plodding tasks and repetitive actions.

They are motivated by appreciation for tasks well done and respond to clear direction. In the referral scenario, they will be agreeable, but not necessarily assertive enough to engage others and convince them to take action. Help your amiables to refer by getting them to bring in or make a connection with someone they could refer, but maneuver into position so you can do the closing to get the best results possible.

These delineations are not intended to judge, but rather to translate your message into a language each kind of person can understand. I learned from Anthony Robbins that there are no resistant people, only inflexible communicators—learn to adapt your approach to the kind of person you are dealing with, and your results will skyrocket, as will their level of satisfaction with you.

Filter 3: Metaprograms

Let's get into the third filter of connection: metaprograms.

I know this is an odd word, but it is an important term in neurolinguistic programming, or NLP.

Metaprograms are generalized, overriding patterns of behavior—in other words, they are tendencies to behave in certain ways in certain situations. There are dozens of such patterns, but we're going to explore three in particular that you will find useful in the referral scenario.

Has this ever happened to you?

You're giving a report of findings, and you explain to the new patient about the many wonderful benefits of chiropractic care. The patient seems unimpressed, claiming to be interested only in getting rid of pain.

Or, while you're presenting your findings, the patient seems to take exception to much of what you say, disagreeing with some of the details.

Or, when you make your recommendations, the patient says, "I need to think about what you've said. I'll call you."

What's wrong with these patients, anyway?

Amazingly, there is nothing defective, resistant, or stupid about these patients. They just need to be communicated with in a particular way, a way that uses their language, their values, and their patterns of behavior.

As a matter of fact, all of these patients probably gave you enough information to be able to communicate with them effectively, if you only knew how to pick up on the clues they left for you. By being sensitive to the typical patterns of someone's behavior, you can anticipate the response and formulate your communication in a way that will work successfully.

We all have our own individual way of processing input, of perceiving what's going on around us, and each of us has a set of patterns of behavior that we use in a given context. These are known as metaprograms.

Metaprograms are often referred to as a sort or filter—in other words, a way of chunking, perceiving, or categorizing something. The first one we'll consider is known as the direction sort, someone's tendency to move toward or away.

Moving Towards Pleasure or Moving Away From Pain

Have you ever noticed that some people tend to be motivated toward pleasure, while others seem to be motivated away from pain? In other words, some may respond to the perceived benefits of a situation, and may be motivated toward them, while others might be impacted more by the potential consequences of a situation, and are motivated away from them. The metaprogram illustrated here is referred to as "direction," and people will tend to use either a moving toward or a moving away pattern.

For example, if in consultation you ask a patient, "What are you look-ing for in a doctor?" the patient could reply, "I'm looking for a doctor who will help me get well, advise me right and care about me." These are examples of benefits the patient desires, so in this context the patient tends to move toward benefits. If, on the other hand, the patient replies to the same question, "I'm looking for a doctor who won't make me wait a long time, who won't rip me off, and who'll get rid of this pain without a lot of fancy doctor talk," this patient is expressing the need to avoid con-sequences, and therefore tends to move away from consequences.

If a patient tends to move toward benefits, choose a communications style that emphasizes the benefits that will be received in your office. For example, you may want to say to the patient, "You are in the right place. You'll find that we really care about our patients, and that we intend to help you get well and stay well. You're going to feel better, your body's going to work better, and you're going to be healthier overall." When you offer positive benefits for these patients to move toward, they feel that you are responsive to their needs, that you are speaking their language.

If a patient tends to move away from consequences, offering positive benefits will not have the same result. Instead, choose a communication style that emphasizes the consequences that they avoid if they follow through with your recommendations. You might say, "You seem like you really want to get rid of this pain. If you're serious about getting this problem fixed, make sure not to miss any appointments, and don't lift anything heavier than ten pounds. You're going to have to avoid anything that could interfere with the healing process, or else your recovery will be delayed."

Now, some of you may be thinking, that's a bit negative, isn't it? Aha! Your metaprograms are showing—someone who tends to move toward will perceive a moving away communication as being negative or unpleasant. On the other hand, someone who tends to move away will perceive a moving toward communication to be uninspiring or unconvincing. Since about half of the population tends to move toward and half tends to move away, it will be very helpful for you to be able to notice who does what, so you can choose language that motivates people effectively and doesn't cost you valuable time and opportunity.

You may be starting to understand why some of your patients seem to follow through on your recommendations and why some don't, though you believe you told them both the same thing. By listening to what people say, and by learning to ask simple questions that give you information about the patient's patterns, you can select the best possible way to communicate, so you and the patient can both get exactly what you want.

Internal or External Frame of Reference

The second pattern we can look at is known as the frame of reference sort, the tendency to have an internal or external frame of reference.

Have you ever had patients listen to your recommendations, and then proceed to do whatever they want anyway? How about the patients who check everything they do with you, just to be sure? These people are demonstrating the metaprogram known as "frame of reference," which has to do with how one evaluates, how one decides if something is true, correct, or good.

Patients who seem to follow their own gut feelings are referred to as internal frame people, and someone who relies more on feedback is called an external frame person.

Try asking the question, "How do you know you've found the right doctor?" An external frame person might say, "I would need an enthusiastic referral from a friend," or maybe, "I always choose doctors by their reputation." To communicate with an external frame person, state your recommendations in an authoritative way, because external people respond well to outside feedback. Say, "I've taken care of many people in your situation, and most have responded beautifully. Just do what I say to do, and avoid the things I tell you not to do, and I expect you to do just great."

On the other hand, an internal frame person, when asked the same question, might say, "I just know," or perhaps, "I get a feeling inside." To communicate with an internal frame person, recognize that any attempts at giving orders or direct commands will not work as well, because this individual is accustomed to trusting internal feelings, not external feedback. Try saying, "You seem like the kind of person who knows what's best for yourself. When you consider the recommendations you're about to hear, you'll probably realize that they are right for you."

Notice that the intention here is not only to persuade the individual that your recommendations are in his or her best interest, but also to respect the person's style of communication and the way he or she interprets reality. Trying to order around an internal frame person is ineffective and confrontational. It makes more sense to select language that really works for both the doctor and the patient, so everybody wins.

Sameness or Differences, Matchers and Mismatchers

The third pattern we'll look at is the relationship sort, the tendency to see the sameness or the differences in things.

How about the patient who seems to be responding beautifully by every method you have of measuring response, and yet complains that "it still hurts"? This patient might also have disagreed with you at different points in your report of findings, picking out details upon which to differ.

On the other side of the same coin, how about the patient who nods in agreement to everything you say? This patient may not really be able to make fine distinctions when you do your testing, stating that it "feels about the same as the other test."

The metaprogram these patients are demonstrating is called "relation-ship," and measures whether someone is more likely to see the same-ness in a relationship, or is more likely to notice the differences in a relationship.

Sameness people, also referred to as matchers, are likely to notice what is the same about things, and to overlook differences. So, if you ask the question, "What was your health like a year ago?" the sameness person may say, "Oh, it's about the same, it's been the same for as long as I can remember."

In contrast, differences people, also known as mismatchers, will probably say, "Oh, it's very different," and proceed to give you a list of details about what specifically is different. The amazing part of this is that they may be describing exactly the same health history—it's just a matter of how they perceive what has happened, based on their patterns of behavior and interpretation.

To communicate with sameness people, show them how things are the same. You might say, "You've probably gotten good results with doctors before, and you can expect to get good results here, too. Your program of care is going to include a series of office visits, most of which will consist of very similar procedures. If we're going to do anything different, I'll make sure to explain everything to you." Interestingly enough, you'll rarely have to explain any differences, because a sameness person will tend to overlook or ignore what is different.

A differences person, on the other hand, will notice anything different, so your best bet is going to be to give the person the opportunity to state whatever differences are detected. You might say, "Today we are going to adjust the second bone in your neck instead of the first one. You may notice that it feels different, so there's no need for concern if it does. By the way, you may find that you feel different afterwards, and if so, it would be completely normal." The differences person will not miss a detail, so letting the individual know that you are aware will ease the patient's mind.

Most people are not pure sameness or pure differences people, but rather tend to notice 'sameness with exceptions' or 'differences with exceptions.' Listen to the way the person communicates, and see if you can recognize these patterns, which may sound like, "It feels almost exactly like the time I hurt myself shoveling snow, except it's a bit lower down into my leg," or, "I've never felt anything like this before, except it's a little like the time I twisted myself swinging a golf club."

The finesse of dealing with people who tend toward sameness revolves around not giving them too many choices or distinctions to make. Say, "You're going to need to come in three times each week for a while, so just stay on that schedule until your next re-examination or until I tell you to change."

In direct opposition, give the person who tends toward differences an obvious choice. "You're going to need daily visits for a while. Which works better for you, mornings or afternoons?" By giving the differences person a detail to decide upon, their tendency to mismatch is satisfied, and then they don't mismatch something you don't want them to mismatch, for example, the necessity for care.

Surprisingly, both sameness and differences people actually want the same outcome—perfection. The distinction is that a differences person will achieve perfection by mismatching every possible detail until things are exactly right, and a sameness person will achieve perfection by overlooking anything that doesn't seem right. They are easy to tell apart because the mismatcher will be much more likely to point out details, especially imperfections. This makes the mismatcher come across as nitpicking, argumentative, or disagreeable, but keep in mind it's only that the person is seeking perfection in his or her own way. Likewise, a matcher may come across as impressionable, gullible, or overly affable. By understanding these behavioral traits, you can decide on the best communication approach for that individual.

What happens if someone is expressing more than one of these patterns at the same time? This is where the skill of using metaprograms in your communication really pays off. If you're talking to an internal frame mismatcher you might say, "Only you know what's best for you, so which works better, mornings or evenings?" Or, you could say to an external frame matcher, "You've got a very similar condition to your friend, Joe, who referred you here, and I expect you to respond just as nicely." Or how about the external frame moving towards matcher, "I bet you noticed how well your friend Mary did in our office, and you want some of the same benefits for yourself." Or perhaps the internal frame moving away mismatcher, "You've probably already figured out that unless you decide to get this problem fixed now by conservative means, you're going to end up choosing between major surgery and a lifetime of chronic pain."

The better you understand the way someone is likely to behave, the better chance you have of communicating effectively with that individual so you both get what you want from your experience together. The three metaprograms we've been discussing are only a few of the many patterns that are being researched.

If you are interested in learning more about metaprograms, pick up a copy of *Unlimited Power* by Anthony Robbins. You may be interested in studying Convincer Strategy, Chunk Size, Time, or many other fascinating behavior patterns.

So, how can we apply these metaprograms specifically in the referral encounter?

Look at the direction sort, the tendency to move toward pleasure or away from pain. When you are eliciting values and gathering leverage, notice if the person responds more to the promise of a better quality of life or the freedom from symptoms and disease. Then, develop leverage by emphasizing the pattern that matches up, keeping in mind that people tend to be blends of the polarities of the metaprograms, based on the shades of variation of emotions and perspectives even within the context of one conversation.

If you are conscious of the frame of reference sort, you can save yourself a lot of unnecessary head banging. If you observe that someone has an external frame of reference, you can use an authority frame, like, "Mrs.

Patient, as an expert in chiropractic pediatrics, it would be my delight to examine your children and confirm their good health." Or, you can use the leverage of social proof, which I learned about in the book *Influence* by Robert Cialdini (see Chapter 4). Social proof means demonstrating validity through common acceptance. You could say, "Mr. Patient, your friend, Joe, recommended you come into our office, and look how good that turned out—who would you like to help in the same way?"

With the relationship sort, you would approach a sameness person by pointing out sameness between their experience in your office and the expected experience of someone they could refer. For example, "Mrs. Patient, you've had a good experience here at Jones Chiropractic, and you can expect that we'll take just as good care of anyone you honor us by referring."

If someone tends to see the differences, though, this comes across as insipid or uninspiring. Instead, say, "Mrs. Patient, you know everyone who gives us the privilege of serving them gets treated like an individual, since everyone needs a different program of care—you can count on us to give the right advice to anyone you send."

Listen to these referral questions, and see if you can pick out the various screens of connection they apply:

Are you the kind of person who shares a good thing with the people you care about, or would you rather just refer someone special to me to take special care of them?

Which would you prefer, to bring the kids in all at once, or one at a time?

Is there any reason why you haven't brought your spouse in to be checked? You do care about his/her health, don't you? Or would you rather wait until something painful and inconvenient happens, like it did to you? Better safe than sorry, wouldn't you say?

As you master these patterns, you'll find that the art of constructing effective referral language is both entertaining and highly productive. For example, for the moving toward external frame matcher, you would say, "In my expert opinion, your great response to our care makes it likely that your children will respond beautifully, too." Or for the moving away internal frame mismatcher, "Only you can understand the consequences of not bringing your wife in for care." These language constructions make your dialogues with patients elegant and highly efficient, and build your reputation and impact as a leader and communicator.

Filter 4: Advanced Personality Type Systems

The final filter of connection is advanced personality type systems, and there are many to be considered—Jung's research, which categorized people as thinkers and feelers, sensors and intuitors, introverts and extraverts, and judgers and perceivers, led to the development of one of the best known personality typing systems, the Myers-Briggs Evaluation.

There is another fascinating field of study, dating back to ancient times, known as *the Enneagram*. It has many applications, one of which is discussing nine basic personality types and using this information as both a tool for better communication and a strategic pathway for growth and enlightenment. (See Resources for *The Enneagram*.)

It's not the purpose of this particular book to cover this advanced material, but rather to alert you to its existence and hopefully inspire you to study it and learn to apply it, as your skill sets deepen and your grasp of communication expands. The more you integrate these advanced techniques, the more positive impact you can have on those you touch and serve.

Listening

You can see that there are many layers of distinctions for you to notice and respond to, but there is a common thread here, and that is the ability to listen. Being a good, engaged listener creates what many refer to as active listening, which means that you are focused on the discourse and paying attention so you can collect and interpret the data available as effectively as possible.

People will expose their values hierarchies, personality tendencies, and beliefs in their conversation, and you can often easily detect the way their system is set up by simply recognizing those details when they talk about them—golf, their grandchildren, gardening, their fears about their health condition, myths and preconceived notions they have picked up along the way—it's all there if you listen for it, and it gives you abundant information to reach them on their terms and skillfully encourage them to act on their own behalf.

Not every exchange between you and a potential patient or referrer goes smoothly, and it would be disingenuous to suggest that it always does. Sometimes, it's as obvious as asking a targeting question that goes wrong—for example, if you ask, "You're married, aren't you?" and the person's face darkens and they say, "Well, yes and no. I'm recently separated..." that would be a time to abort the mission. Extricate yourself by acknowledging the inadvertent foot in mouth and say, "It seems I've opened a can of worms without realizing it, please forgive me. I was only going to offer to help your family, but it doesn't seem appropriate to discuss that right now."

The patient will usually forgive the transgression and make it okay based on the apology, and they either will or will not want to continue the conversation—take their lead, and go from there.

That's why this is not just about learning scripting—you must keep your outcome in mind, and if it looks like you will not be able to get there, cut your losses quickly and salvage the relationship with the patient.

Overcoming Objections

There is a well-known language construction that eases you through objections, usually referred to as "feel, felt, found." It's used when someone raises an objection, like time, money, or distance. You would simply apply the three words in order—"You know, I'm not surprised you feel that way. In fact, I've felt that way myself at times, and you know what I found?" Then, you address the objection.

For example, let's say it's an objection based on the cost of your care. You could say, "I can appreciate how you feel. In fact, I've felt that way myself at times, but you know what I found? Making this investment in your health actually saves you money, not to mention inconvenience and suffering. Taking care of this now before it gets too bad actually costs less in the long run."

Or, let's say it's a matter of time—"My husband would come in, but he's too busy." You could respond, "I can respect how he feels—many patients have felt that way, but you know what they found? By making time now, they avoided the inconvenience of having a poorly timed flare-up or acute attack, which would pull much more time out of his schedule than taking care of it now."

These are simple reframes that work in a practical setting—try them and see.

When you begin to use these tools, you will at times be rejected bluntly, usually not viciously, but some people will bat you away no matter how skillful you become at overcoming objections. You can also expect some people to embrace you and your message enthusiastically. This is true of everyone, no matter the skill or experience level. But the point is, you'll need to make enough attempts at this to get good at it, and that means you're going to get some rejection.

If you think they are rejecting you personally, it will hurt and make you not want to do it.

But they're almost never rejecting you personally. They are not in a position to fully understand your message, and you can't be responsible for what they do or don't do. You can only become as skillful and polished as possible at engaging them and inviting them into your world, and the rest is up to them.

The Five SWs

It's like the Five SWs—some will... some won't... so what? Someone's waiting—spread the word!

This brings Chapter 2 on the referral process to a close. Study these tools and you will dramatically increase the number of referrals you attract, up to the level of your current capacity. Some doctors attract new patients every day just through referral!

If you use these techniques and they work well for you, congratulations on helping more people! If not, you can check to see if you have enough capacity to accept more new patients, and if not, look in Chapter 1 for some tools to increase your capacity or attraction.

Points to Remember

1. Before asking for a referral, know your outcome and gain rapport.

2. The referral process has three parts—target the potential referral, gain leverage by asking values-driven questions, and close effectively.

3. Invest the time and energy to learn whom you are dealing with—be a great listener, and use what you learn to connect.

Actions to Take

1. Role-play common referral scenarios with your team and/or colleagues to improve your skill and gather experiences to refine your approach.

2. Practice overcoming common objections in staff meetings or special masterminds.

3. Play the three-a-day game for a month in your office, and see how your results compare to the same month last year.

Questions to Ponder

1. What percentage of your new patients come through referrals? Is that satisfying for you? How could you increase your referrals?

2. Are referral patients more or less compliant than people who find you other ways?

Now that you have a foundation in the art of the one-on-one referral encounter, you can begin to expand your outreach. In Chapter 3 we'll explore how to network with local professionals, applying the ideas and systems we've developed in these first two chapters.

CHAPTER 3

Networking With Professionals

When I was in practice, I took care of a lot of children, and some of them had learning problems, a group I was often able to help. I remember a young lady named Veronica, about twelve years old, whose whole family came in for care—she had learning issues, and regularly attended a learning center in my town. When she started to respond to our care, she drew a picture of our office and wrote the word *chiropractor* on the front window, with all the letters facing correctly. When she showed the drawing around at the learning center, the director saw it and gave me a call to find out what I was doing.

That phone call resulted in about one new patient each month for the next eight years, about a hundred patients or so, adding up to about a quarter of a million dollars from that one phone call.

One of the richest resources you can find to generate a steady flow of new people into your practice is the network of other local professionals who provide your ideal patients with other services and products you don't offer. They are not your competition—they are your allies, if you know how to create the right kind of relationship with them. This chapter is about how to do that effectively.

As many of you know, my dad, may he rest in peace, was also a chiropractor. Along with a couple of partners, he built one of the largest personal injury practices in south Florida history. They had about ten offices going at their peak, and engaged the legal profession at the highest level to feed their offices.

For example, one year they flew a bunch of their favorite attorneys out to the NBA All-Star game, furnished them with beautiful NBA leather jackets, and entertained them for the weekend. Over the top, you might think? Perhaps, but it set them apart from others trying to woo them, and the effort turned into millions in personal injury cases they might not have gotten any other way.

The point is, you need to know your patient, and you also need to know the professionals who could be referring you patients. We're going to examine this kind of relationship building in a few minutes.

But first, let's dig deeper into the foundations of referral technique to pick up some pointers before we launch ourselves at these local professionals.

One-On-One Marketing Skills

How many new patients do you need to build the practice of your dreams—five per week, ten, twenty? Now, think about all the people you come in contact with each week who are not your patients. Many of these people can be your patients if you use certain communication skills. The purpose of this section is to give you some techniques for one-on-one marketing. As usual, there are two preliminary steps before you enter into any conversation with a prospective patient.

Prepare Yourself First

First, prepare yourself for what you're about to do. Think about your outcome. Say to yourself, "What is it that I want to accomplish here?" This will focus you on your target, in this case, to get this individual motivated to become your patient.

Second, make sure you are ready to enter into this kind of situation. You must be prepared physically and mentally, and that means that as you focus on your outcome, ask yourself, "What is the best way for me to show up right now to get this person motivated to become my patient? How can I connect? Should I be enthusiastic and compassionate? Smooth and professional? Casual and friendly?"

Notice that you are capable of a wide variety of approaches, so choose the one you believe will work best with this particular person. Another way to say this is to get yourself into the right state. Your state simply means what you are doing with your mind and body at that particular time. Make sure that your state and the resources you have available match up with your outcome, and then the stage is set to begin your one-on-one marketing techniques.

Get Leverage

Think for a moment; what would make this prospect want to become your patient? It really boils down to one thing—the patient must see the value. This person, like everyone else (including you), has a million things to do every day and dozens of people soliciting him or her with causes they believe in. This person must quickly evaluate whether your solicitation is any more important than the others, because only the most important things get attention.

Therefore, if you try to reposition the person to align with what's important to you, your batting average will suffer and, indeed, this is why most salespeople of all kinds have such trouble selling—because they are trying to sell based on *their own* values instead of the obvious and superior alternative, which is of course to sell based on the *prospect's* values. In fact, it's a lot harder to sell someone something than to inspire them to buy it.

In other words, motivate the person by showing that something that is already important to him or her would be served by becoming your patient.

When you demonstrate to prospects that their best interests are supported by your service, they're motivated to become patients because they understand what's in it for them.

Find Out What's Important to the Other Person

So, how do you find out what's important to someone? Often, you can tell what someone cares about by listening to the content and emphasis in his or her conversation. If someone is constantly talking about tennis, or about his boat, or about her children, or about their work, you can be sure this is something that is important to the person. Use this to develop leverage.

This means helping them see how being your patient actually helps them with their values.

For example, let's say you're at a party and you hear somebody talking about how much he enjoys playing tennis. He's playing twice a week and is starting to get more serious about his game. When the time is right, approach him and say, "I couldn't help overhearing how important your tennis game is to you."

He'll respond, "Yeah, I really love to play," and then you can begin to steer the conversation by asking a question—"If there was something you could do that might give you an advantage that can help you play better, would you be interested?"

If tennis is really important to him, as you have already qualified, then he'll say, "Of course, I want any edge I can get!"

Then you can say, "Most people don't realize how important spinal movement is to the tennis stroke and serve. They think about their arms and legs, but without flexible spinal motion, power is lost and range is diminished. My patients who are tennis players tell me that since they have been taking better care of their structure, they can serve harder and reach deeper into their backhands, and their overall game is much improved. If you are as serious about your game as you seem, it might be wise for you to get your spine checked by a specialist. Tell me, what neighborhood do you live in?"

If the patient says somewhere too far to come to your office, then, if you can, make a referral right there. Use a long-handled spoon—believe me, it will come back to you many times over.

Or, if the patient says, "Well, I live right here in town," then you can say, "Hey, that's really close to my office. If you feel okay about us meeting under these circumstances, you know, at a party and everything, then it would be a pleasure to examine you and make some recommendations. If for any reason you don't feel comfortable with that, I will be glad to help you pick someone else here in town."

The person will usually say, "Oh, no, I don't want to go to someone else, I'd rather just come to you" and bam! You just got a new patient, it's as simple as that.

Did we talk about the value of lifetime chiropractic care? Did we talk about hard bones on soft nerves? Did we talk about the politics of health care? Absolutely not, because those things are important to you, but not to the prospect.

When you stick with the prospect's values, you have a much better chance of getting through. This kind of approach is very flexible and can be adapted to almost any situation. Remember it when we start to address networking with professionals.

For example, let's say you're waiting in line at the bank (not the most exciting part of your day), and as fate would have it, you happen to be standing behind a young woman with a five-year-old boy hanging onto her leg. You can stand there like a lump or you can use the time and opportunity to your advantage.

Break the ice with a compliment, "What a handsome son you have there." She will smile and say thanks.

You can continue, "I can tell he really loves you and it seems you are pretty crazy about him, too." She'll smile again and you can continue, "I'll bet that, like all concerned parents, you really want the best for him, don't you? I mean, you want him to grow up healthy and happy, right?"

She'll say, "Of course, I do."

Then you can say, "So, if there was something that might be harmful to him, you'd want to find out about it and take care of it, wouldn't you?"

At this point, her eyes will narrow and she may say, "What do you mean" or just look at you quizzically.

Then you smile and say, "Don't worry, Mom, it's just that I really love kids too, and I hate the thought of a child suffering needlessly or growing up with problems that should have been dealt with while he was young. I am Dr. Perman, and I help people get well and stay well naturally. I couldn't help noticing that your son is putting his weight more on his left side instead of being balanced on both legs, and sometimes that means there is the beginning of a problem there. Tell me, when was the last time you had his structure and his nerve system evaluated?"

Most of the time she'll say, "Well, never," or, "I don't really know," or, "Oh, his pediatrician probably does that."

You can reply, "You know, I am not surprised that you're not so aware of the importance of keeping your brain, nerve system, and spine healthy, since it's only recently that people are learning how important it is. Nevertheless, if you really care about your child's health, as I'm sure you do, you may want to arrange for an examination. Tell me, what neighborhood do you live in?" Bam! New patient!

See how I resisted the impulse to spew my philosophy all over her? She is interested in what's important to her, and my challenge is to put my message in terms she can instantly relate to.

I remember a time when I was sitting in a restaurant and as I read my menu the server came over and said, "What'll it be?"

I said, "Well, I'd like to start with a bowl of vegetable soup," and she wrote it down. Then I said, "And, I think I'd also like a grilled cheese sandwich." As I looked up from the menu, I stared briefly at her shoulders and said, "Did you know that your left shoulder is higher than your right?"

She said, "What?"

I said, "Gee, I didn't mean to offend you, please let me introduce myself. I am Dr. Dennis Perman, and I help people get healthier by reducing stress on their brain, nerve system, and spine. I noticed some signs of such stress in you, so would it be okay if I asked you a few questions?"

She said yes, and I continued, "I noticed some distortion in your spine. Tell me, do you stand on your feet all day?"

Now, I know she does, because all servers do, and true to form she said, "Yes, I do."

I said, "Do you usually carry your tray on one side rather than the other?" knowing full well she does, because pretty much all servers do.

She said, "Well, yes."

I said, "Which side do you usually carry your tray on?"

She said, "The left."

I said, "Are you right-handed or left-handed?"

She said, "Right-handed."

I said, "Hmm, I thought so—can I have that grilled cheese on whole wheat bread?"

She said, "Forget your lunch, pal—what about my shoulders?" At this point, I had her full attention.

I said, "Look, at the end of a day, do you feel tired and stiff in your upper back and neck?"

She said, "You're darned right I do!"

I said, "We should really get that checked out, because if you don't, it's probably going to get slowly worse until it interferes with your work, not to mention the rest of your life. Tell me, what neighborhood do you live in?" Bam! New patient!

Did you pick up on how many questions I asked? By asking questions, I control the communication. Also, I phrased my questions so that they could be answered with a "yes" response. When I get the person saying yes to small commitments, I have a better shot of getting a yes on a big commitment. This communications tool will be explained in more detail in Chapter 4.

Remember to Keep Rapport

Remember to keep rapport throughout the interaction. Keep your connection with the person by using a comfortable pace, tonality, and posture so the person feels a bond with you while you are speaking.

Above all, remember that people will be motivated to take action only by what they perceive is important to them. People will move towards things they find pleasurable and away from things they find painful. If you're going to get a patient to choose you and chiropractic, you'll have to get leverage based on the benefits and consequences as perceived by the prospect.

Show someone how it's good to be your patient and bad not to be your patient, and these one-on-one marketing techniques will bring you all the new patients you can possibly want.

Let's look at one more hands-on technique before we start applying these tools directly to professional referrals. To me, this is the best story-of-the-day scripting.

The Best Story of the Day Scripting

If you want to help as many people as possible, then you are probably always on the lookout for convenient and productive ways to attract more new patients. Over the years, I've noticed that if a technique is cost-effective and time-effective, then it's more likely that a doctor will choose it and use it.

Busy doctors need tools to increase patient flow that won't cost a lot of time or money, and one of the best methods I know that fits these criteria is referred to as "story of the day."

Story of the day is one way you can give your patients lots of information and also encourage them to refer their friends and family. Story of the day can be one of your most powerful in-office referral tools, because it serves the dual purpose of letting your patients know that you are available to help others, and also reminding them of people they know whom they can refer.

Story of the day scripting can be delivered from either of two perspectives, depending on your practice orientation and the particular patient you are talking to.

If your practice is a wellness-oriented practice, then you can use a wellness-oriented story of the day script. Or, if your practice also includes pain relief in dealing with conditions, then you can also use a condition-oriented story of the day.

All You Need is Five Simple Lines

For example, let's say that in your practice you do deal with painful problems and you'd like to attract more people with painful problems so you can help them. Along comes Mr. Patient who is suffering from low back pain, and has been doing very nicely under your care.

After you greet him and he makes a few comments about how he is doing, he lies down on the adjusting table. Part of the beauty of story of the day is that it can be done while the patient is on the table, so it takes no additional time.

Put your hands on his back so you feel the rate of his breathing and speak at the same rate. This creates an excellent rapport between you. Base your story on a condition that is not the condition this patient has suffered from. He already knows you can help people with that problem. This story will broaden his understanding so he can send other people with varying conditions.

Open your script with a question like, "The most amazing thing happened to me today. Do you want to hear about it?" The patient will say yes, (or actually more like "ymph" because his face is in the headrest paper. This is okay because you really don't want much feedback until the end anyway.)

Now that you have his attention and his permission to continue, you can proceed with your story. "Well, this lady came in for her adjustment today. She has been a patient here for about four weeks, and you know, she has been suffering with these terrible migraine headaches for over ten years. Do you know what she told me today? She hasn't had a headache all week, and it's the first time in ten years she's gone a week without a headache. Isn't that amazing?"

Pause for just a moment, not to get a response, but just to give the patient time to think about what you just said and integrate it. Then you can continue. "You know, I wish more people realized how great chiropractic care is for people with headache problems."

Once again, pause for a moment to let the person think and integrate, then you can continue. "You know, I bet that even you know someone who is suffering needlessly from headaches who can really be helped by chiropractic."

Now at this point, many people will jump in and say, "Gee, Doc, now that you mention it, my neighbor gets these really bad headaches and she has to go to bed for a day with a damp rag over her face until it goes away."

Then you can reply, "Well, then, I'm really glad I brought it up. What do you think is the best way to get your neighbor the help she needs? Do you want to bring her the next time you come in, or do you think it would be better for us to call her directly on your behalf and set up a convenient time for her to come in?"

This scripting has stimulated many, many chiropractic patients to make referrals, so let's take a few moments to explore why this approach is so effective.

Why This Works

The first reason this works is that you are creating a good connection with the person you are asking for the referral. Who has more confidence in you than a patient who is responding well? Plus, you have added the advantage of talking at the rate the patient is breathing, creating a deep physiological rapport.

Secondly, you are getting permission from the patient to tell your story. By obtaining consent from the patient, there is an implicit agreement to participate, and this increases your batting average. And your enthusiasm makes it unlikely that the patient will withhold that consent. He or she is going to want to know about your amazing experience.

Thirdly, you are talking about a condition the patient doesn't have, and therefore, never really thought about. By changing the patient's focus and perspective to a new condition, an assortment of new potential referrals comes into his or her mind. Then, you have a chance to ask if he or she knows anybody who has been suffering needlessly, and often a response just pops out, because you have skillfully and articulately guided the patient's thinking in this direction.

Finally, in your closing, you do what effective closers tell you to do—you offer a choice between two alternatives that are good for you, good for the referral, and good for the referrer as well. Using this win-win-win approach, your efforts are correctly considered as genuine and compassionate, not hungry and manipulative. Remember, when you offer your services to people, you may be doing them the greatest favor of their lives, sparing them unnecessary pain and suffering and exposing them to some new information that can help them and their loved ones have a better life.

Use This Variation for Wellness Patients

The story of the day script we just developed works great in practices that talk about pain, symptoms, and conditions, and can bring you many, many additional referrals.

But, what if your practice is more wellness-oriented, and you prefer to attract health-oriented clientele rather than patients requiring a lot of relief-oriented care? Here is a version of the same kind of story of the day script delivered with the same effective language constructions, but from a wellness perspective.

Once again, the patient is face down, a captive audience, and you can gain rapport by placing your hands on his or her back and speaking at the same rate as his or her breathing. Once again, you can open with the same line, "The most amazing thing happened today. Do you want to hear about it?"

The patient says ymph and you can continue. "Well, this guy called up today and said that he wanted to begin his care here as a patient, and the amazing thing was, he doesn't have any complaints, problems or pain— he just heard from his friends that chiropractic care is really good for you and he wants to be as healthy as possible. Isn't that amazing?"

Pause for a moment to give the patient a chance to think and integrate. Then you can continue, "You know, I really wish more people realized how great chiropractic care is for your body just as health care, that you don't need a painful problem to really benefit from chiropractic."

Once again, pause for a moment to give the patient a chance to think and integrate. Then you can say, "You know, I'll bet that you know someone who is really into health and taking care of his or her body who would want chiropractic care as part of their normal health routine if they knew about it."

At this point, many patients will say, "Gee, now that you mention it, Doc, my brother is really into health. He runs every day and is always talking about taking good care of himself," or, "Now that you mention it, my neighbor is really into health. She is always talking about eating right and bothering my husband to quit smoking."

You can say, "Well, I'm glad I brought it up. What do you think is the best way to get her the information she needs? Would she want to come with you next time you come in, or do you think she'd prefer to attend our health talk and find out firsthand more about what we do here?"

Notice once again that the closing offers a choice, this time between coming with the referrer or attending a health talk. Other possible options could include a complimentary consultation or an invitation to a promotional event. After a patient mentions a prospective referral, make a note on the patient's record so you can follow up on the lead. Also, make a note on the record that you've done that particular script, so patients don't hear the same story over again, and also so you can follow up if appropriate to do so.

You can do this technique at least two days out of each month and if you run out of amazing stories of your own, borrow some from your colleagues and friends. Just change the script to, "I was talking with a friend of mine who is also a chiropractor and he told me the most amazing story. Do you want to hear about it?"

Practice getting your story of the day techniques smooth and natural sounding. The power of this approach is in the conversational attitude, so make it just like telling a story and you will find it extremely productive.

Doctors who tell story of the day on a regular basis can expect more referrals and a better-educated patient who is more aware of the often miraculous benefits of chiropractic care.

Now that we've covered all these referral tools, let's see how we can turn them into a steady stream of referrals from your neighboring professionals.

Creating Professional Inter-Referral Relationships

Now we're going to consider the values, beliefs, and behaviors of typical professionals in your neighborhood that could be good candidates for your inter-referral network.

Medical practitioners learned long ago the art of interdisciplinary referral, or referral to a doctor in another specialty. They have formed networks of various practitioner specialists with whom they can inter-refer patients. To them, it means ongoing referrals from a perpetual source; patients coming into a funnel and being routed within the network to maximize the benefit to the patient and include specialists in their areas of expertise. All practitioners in the network act as a source of potential referrals, and each doctor learns how to use the services of network colleagues to make sensible and relevant referrals.

Unfortunately, doctors of chiropractic seem to have been left out of the referral algorithm, meaning that physicians who practice traditional medicine have not been taught to refer—at least, their neuro-musculo-skeletal cases, and at best, those patients seeking proactive advice on the wellness lifestyle—to chiropractors. Once again, it is a job of education that unfortunately must be handled by the individual DC.

Please note that it is not necessary to educate every doctor you know as to the wonders of chiropractic. Many won't believe you anyway! Be patient and flexible, and let the process unfold. It is, however, your job to subtly teach them who, when, and how to refer to a chiropractor ... more specifically, to you!

Here is a proven procedure that works in establishing a reputation with allied practitioners in a given neighborhood.

Send a Consultation Note

1. At the end of the consultation, ask the patient's permission to send a consultation note to his/her family physician. Most patients will be appreciative, while some may prefer that you refrain from notifying their doctor, fearing conflict. In that case, it is best to comply with the patient's wishes. But barring resistance, communicate with the patient's other doctors.

2. Send a consultation note with a cover letter something like this:

Dear Dr. Smith:

Your patient, Mr. Patient, presented himself at our office today seeking consultation with regard to a lower back syndrome. As he named you as his personal family physician, I thought you'd appreciate a copy of my consultation notes, so your own records will reflect this incident.

I would be happy to forward a complete narrative upon your request, and have taken the liberty of enclosing my curriculum vitae for your inspection.

Should you have any questions regarding this matter, please do not hesitate to call me personally.

Sincerely,
Your name, DC.

It is important to follow the above-described procedure with a telephone call. Simply say that you are calling to introduce yourself and ask if he/she received your note. Then ask if he/she has any established relationships with other chiropractors. Follow that question by asking if he/she thinks it is worth a "get acquainted" lunch to determine if you have the basis for reciprocal referral.

They may or may not want to do so, so go easy, and maybe the second or third time, they'll be more open to it. If you do this consistently, before you know it you will start to gain a positive reputation from the doctors you contact.

In fact, you'd be surprised how often your name will come up in their conversations. When asked by other colleagues, their personal acquaintances, or even their own patients what they think of chiropractic, they even start to brag that they know a great chiropractor. It seems to be a badge of honor or a method of displaying how modern they are.

Nevertheless, sooner or later, this action step will become a new source of referrals to your office. Look for opportunities to nurture these young professional relationships, and they will bear fruit as they mature.

Building Relationships with Medical Doctors

The first time you engage a local MD who takes care of your patient, it is probably too early to begin to solicit referrals in this first exposure to you. But the second time you send a consultation note to a particular local MD, you can begin to broach the subject. You can add a PS on the note: "By the way, Dr. Smith, it seems that several of my patients enjoy your services. Perhaps we should meet so we have a chance to compare notes and better help our mutual patients."

Then, just leave it at that at first—you can wait to see if the doctor expresses interest, or you can contact him or her a week or two later by phone to see if you can arrange for a lunch date, coffee, or a tour of one or both of your offices. This will generate a subtle connection between you two, which develops at a rate that is consistent with the other professional's pace.

Not every MD will be interested in meeting with you, but some may be. For those who are, aim for a dignified, elegant tone to your early engagement, until you learn more about the style of the particular doctor. Match your tone to theirs the best you can to generate early rapport and an inviting atmosphere.

Often, the receptionist or assistant is trained not to let calls through to the doctor, but if you identify yourself as a doctor as well, you have a better chance. Whoever answers the phone in a medical office is usually busy, so cut to the chase. If the CA calls for you, the receptionist will probably answer with "Doctor Smith's office" and your CA can say, "Hello, my name is Susie, calling on behalf of Dr. Jones. Who am I speaking with?" Always get a name so you have someone in the office you can ask for. Then, use the person's name as you talk, to make the conversation more personal.

"Mary, Dr. Jones had a patient of Dr. Smith's come in, and he'd like to speak with Dr. Smith about that—when would be a good time for them to talk?"

If your assistant has trouble getting through, you may need to make the call yourself, and the likelihood of connecting will go up.

If there are no patients in common and it's more of a cold call, you can still connect with the doctor by finding out a little about his or her practice, so you have a sense of which patients you could refer that fall within the doctor's specialty.

Let's say you are able to arrange a luncheon date with a local internist. Meet at a neighborhood restaurant to demonstrate that you are a community-minded professional. Get there early, and plan to pick up the tab. Let the restaurant know it's an important meeting, and you'd like a quiet table so you can talk.

When the doctor arrives, you should already be at the restaurant, and you should be standing when you greet your guest warmly. Move to the table together, and let him or her choose a seat first. You want the doctor to be as comfortable as possible, and to read you as a friendly and cooperative person.

Start building rapport immediately with matching and mirroring, and if the doctor gives you cues like word choices, pace, or tonality, give back those detectable characteristics to generate connection.

Keep your outcome clearly in mind as you begin the conversation—thank you for coming, I've been looking forward to meeting you, please tell me a little about yourself and your practice. Ask open probe questions designed to elicit your prospect's values as a person and as a professional.

"How long have you practiced in Anytown? What do you like best about practicing here? What would you change if you could? What kind of patients do you focus on? Who are your favorite patients to take care of? Who are your biggest challenges?"

Gather distinctions about your guest's values by asking questions about his or her practice. Listen carefully and actively, asking questions along the way to learn as much as possible.

This does two things—firstly, it gives you information you can use later to cement your relationship and set the stage for inter-referral. Secondly, you'd be talking about your guest's most enjoyable topic of conversation—him or herself. It makes you seem like better company if you follow Stephen Covey's advice—first understand, then seek to be understood.

At this point, everything inside of you wants to even the score and download your details to your guest, but unless invited, resist the impulse to spew all over him or her. Be patient and wait—you will probably get your chance, but even if you don't, you will have made great progress at creating a relationship with this doctor, and that is a necessary precondition to having any luck at all with inter-referral.

If you do get an opportunity to share some of your information, do it concisely, and match your tone to that of your guest. You can be enthusiastic and passionate, just don't rave, because in that setting it comes across as hard sell. Be gently strong, authentic, and certain of your sense of self, and you will connect better.

Engage on common values. "Like you, Doctor, I focus on young families," or "I'm not surprised to see your enthusiasm about treating your patients—that's something we share."

Find out what's important to the doctor. Don't assume your problems and theirs overlap, or that what would fulfill you in practice is similar for them. Many MDs have more than enough new patients, so they are less interested in referrals than you might be. In fact, for these doctors, you would do them a favor by being able to take some of their difficult patients off their hands. "Say, Doc, if you don't like taking care of those tough low back pain patients, I work with them all the time; maybe I could lighten your load."

You can use the story of the day format, or the target, leverage, close format, depending on which seems to fit better.

For example, you could use the story of the day format because it's conversational, and as my dear partner Dr. Bob Hoffman teaches, facts are forgotten, but stories are remembered and retold.

If you have worked at developing a relationship, both through gaining rapport and eliciting and supporting values, and the types of patients they like and don't like, you will probably have the opportunity to say, "Hey, Doc, something interesting happened in my office, do you wanna hear about it? This woman came into my office with such and such a problem, and today she told me she's doing so much better. I bet you didn't realize we take care of people with such and such. You know, if you have patients with such and such, you may want to let me take a look—if

I can help them, I'll help them and then send them back to you, and if not, I'll just send them right back to you."

Medical doctors are accustomed to referring according to specialty—if they don't know where you fall in the referral algorithm, they don't know how to send you people. You must define it for them, once you have heard them out and they have invited you to tell them what you do.

Remember that they may not speak your language, so be careful not to overstate your case. Stay in your sweet spot, whatever that is—if you feel confident discussing the finer points of neurology, that's fine, but remember that your guest has a well-developed network for those patients that are perceived to be beyond their neurological knowledge. That doesn't mean you should be relegated to a back pain mechanic, but bring your new relationship along at a reasonable pace—it took you a while to develop your deeper understanding of chiropractic philosophy, so you'll do better to allow such a process in your professional network.

Like any other relationship, it may take some time before you can move forward as you wish. Be patient, let the process unfold, and you're better off not pushing too hard—discretion is the better part of valor here, and if you don't mess it up, you'll have time to nurture the relationship and turn it into more people to help, even if it takes a bit longer than you expected.

Medical specialists may be easier to engage than internists or general surgeons. Consider patients you love taking care of, and which professionals have patients like that you could serve. If you want more kids, engage pediatricians and OB/GYNs. If you like seniors, try a gerontologist, a cardiologist, or a rheumatologist.

If you are a generalist, as most chiropractors tend to be, dentists, psychologists, podiatrists, and dermatologists make good referral partners, as there is little overlap between their work and yours. All of your people will need some dental care, and all of your dentist's patients will need some chiropractic, so these relationships are natural and easy to form.

If you have a specialty practice, like ART, extremity adjusting, nutrition, or sports, for example, use your creativity to establish connections with a variety of relevant professionals—sports doctors, physical therapists, physiatrists, orthopedists, and neurologists can be open to sending you their tough cases. Once you earn their confidence, they will often use you as a first-thought referral and not only as a last resort, especially when you find patients in their sweet spots and refer them appropriately. This is the holy grail of medical referrals, having parity in their minds and inspiring them to insert you into their personal referral algorithm.

Building Relationships with Attorneys

Now, let's turn our attention toward attorneys, for those who would like to increase their personal injury referrals. Lawyers notoriously refer to professionals they like, so befriending attorneys you'd like to work with is a good first step.

You don't need to go overboard, like when you're marketing a major personal injury chain. But you do need to be prepared, both logistically, and also by becoming aware of the lawyer's key values around working with someone like you.

The attorney wants a good settlement, both for the client, and because that's how they get paid, so anything you do that makes a smooth and easy path to settlement is good, and anything that interferes with quick resolution is bad. Your challenge is to show attorneys that what you do can help them to accomplish what they already want.

Ask the attorney questions about what he or she looks for in experts to work with—if you want to work with personal injury patients, you must be willing to prepare yourself in the ways that support a legal case—documentation, proper terminology, and a commitment to be timely with your reporting are basic standards that make a lawyer want to work with you. Act like you've been there, even if in the beginning you have to feel your way. Again, keep your outcome in mind, and gain rapport with the attorney—it sets the stage for you to make the encounters productive, even if it takes a few attempts to get something going.

Prove yourself to be reliable—do your paperwork on a timely basis, prepare thoroughly if you need to testify, and above all, treat the attorney with respect. If you say you're going to do something, do it—and you'll get more referrals, because attorneys will feel like they can count on you, both to make their cases easier, and to avoid being held up by someone less responsible than you.

For example, you could use a target, leverage, close format when speaking with an attorney. "Mr. Lawyer, do you have clients who were injured in auto accidents? Did you know that some chiropractors specialize in the long-term effects of soft tissue and nerve injuries, with or without fracture? If we could help some of those clients you thought were borderline to get reasonable settlements for their suffering by effectively describing the real damage done, would you be curious enough to send me a patient or two to see how we work together?"

Building Relationships with other Chiropractors

Another group of professionals you can inter-refer with are... other chiropractors. There are two broad categories of DCs you can inter-refer with; doctors in different locations, and doctors with different specialties.

Remember the long-handled spoons—if a patient comes in to see you who would be better served elsewhere, have the courage and kindness to make a referral to another chiropractor. I did this many times, and the relationships that were created generated at least as many patients in return, most of whom were a better fit with me than the ones I sent out.

Develop a file of chiropractors in various places, starting with friends and classmates, and then extending to those DCs you meet when making a referral to a location other than your town, to make the patient's chiropractic experience more geographically desirable.

The other type of intra-chiropractic referral is to a chiropractic specialist, like a chiropractic pediatrician, functional neurologist, or an expert in a particular technique, like extremities, instrument adjusting, or cranial work. Again, develop a list of doctors in your area who focus on various chiropractic subspecialties to better serve your patients and open the channels of cooperation between you and the other chiropractors in your area, who are more like teammates than competition.

If you believe that we live in a friendly, abundant universe, then you can refer your patients to other chiropractors without fear or doubt. The number of patients you see is dependent more on your capacity and attraction than on the available pool of new patients, which is for all intents and purposes, unlimited.

The Patient-Centered Medical Home: The New Professional Network

There's one more major area where developing an inter-referral network will play an integral role, and that is in the formation of the Patient-Centered Medical Home, or PCMH, which is the basic unit of health care delivery in the Affordable Care Act. No matter where you stand on health care reform, this is a tremendous opportunity for chiropractors, so let me explain a little about the PCMH model and what it has to do with increasing your professional referrals.

I first heard about this novel idea from Dr. Gerry Clum, and when I started to understand it, my mouth hung open. It seems that while doctors have traditionally been paid for time and services rendered, the Affordable Care Act shifts the focus to outcomes—doctors are paid for their outcomes. That means that keeping someone well and/or getting them well as efficiently as possible affects the bottom line directly.

So, the patient-centered medical home, a fancy phrase for a doctor's group practice or network, accepts patients and works with them to get the best outcome possible as quickly and as inexpensively as possible. Doctors who want to maximize the system will have to develop networks of doctors of different fields of study to team up on behalf of the patient.

You may do this anyway, but there's a special incentive built into the system, and here's how I understand it to work.

When a patient comes to you or one of the doctors in your PCMH, the insurance carrier receives an original claim form and assigns a value to the case based on what they have paid for cases with the same diagnosis in the past. That's one reason it's a bad idea to minimize or down-code a patient's condition, or to erroneously use a lesser diagnosis—the insurance company expects to have to pay a certain amount based on the diagnosis, and if the program of care doesn't match up, they object.

In the old system, the doctor submitted the diagnosis, the carrier put aside that amount of money, and if they didn't spend it all on the patient's care, they kept the difference.

Now here's the amazing opportunity built into the Affordable Care Act. If you and your network get better results than expected, costing less than expected, the insurance carrier will split the difference with you. In other words, if a low back patient comes to your network and the carrier puts aside $50,000 in anticipation of eventual surgery and rehabilitation, and you help the patient with $4,000 of chiropractic care and save the patient from surgery, the carrier will split the money they saved with your network—in this case, half of $46,000, or $23,000 to your network. Multiply that by great results with many patients, and it turns into serious money!

Using The Masters Circle App as a Resource

So, it is worth it to develop relationships with local professionals who will be part of your inter-referral network both between you, and also as part of a patient-centered medical home. If you want to know more about health care reform for chiropractors, download The Masters Circle app onto your phone or tablet, and click on the teleseries button.

Then just scroll down to the teleclass called Health Care Reform 101, and you'll have a 45-minute class with Dr. Hoffman and Dr. Clum about the way chiropractors can capitalize on the Affordable Care Act and the PCMH model. It is perhaps the greatest opportunity for networking with other local professionals ever available.

The Masters Circle app has dozens of free teleclasses and other useful content, so please check it out.

It's About Capacity and Attraction

Remember to apply the basic principles we have covered in the first two chapters when working with other professionals. First, make sure you have sufficient capacity to handle what you set out to accomplish. Do you have enough help to make your calls, schedule your appointments, serve that kind of patient, or do you need to add hands?

Are your days and hours in alignment with the kinds of patients you are seeking? Are you moving quickly enough in the right direction? Do you have the systems, the scripting, the training, the equipment, the paperwork, and all the components you'll need?

Are you generating attraction by riding the interface between being and doing, by bringing great energy to optimal habits, like getting your paperwork done, nurturing your professional relationships, or sending consultation notes and thank you notes?

Remember to gain and maintain rapport, and to sculpt your conversation around the other party's values. Showing the other person how doing what you want helps them get something they want is the shortest distance between you and the referrals you desire.

Networking with professionals is cumulative—as you develop and enrich the relationships you create, the number of local professionals who know you, respect you, and refer to you, increases. If you have one doctor or lawyer sending you one new patient a month, then you get, well, one new patient a month from your network. But if you have a dozen or more professionals sending you one or two new patients each month, out of the hundreds of professionals within striking distance of most neighborhoods, you could end up with new patients every day just from your professional referrals.

As you start to collect more and more new patient attraction strategies, try them on for size—some will fit better than others. But the only way for you to discover what works for you is to put the technique in play and see what happens. Every one of these tools works, up to the level of your own capacity and your ability to fill it with attraction.

Points to Remember

3. As in any referral scenario, you need to develop a relationship with professionals in your sphere of influence by gaining rapport and eliciting values.

4. By understanding what's in it for them, you can develop win-win relationships with your professional neighbors.

Actions to Take

1. Target three local professionals—one medical doctor, one attorney, and one chiropractor, and create three strategies to connect with them and initiate a referral relationship.

2. Learn about the changes in the health care laws and study how you can make them work for you and your patients.

Questions to Ponder

1. What would happen if more doctors worked together to serve our communities?

2. What would it be worth to you and your practice to attract one more professional referral each week?

This concludes the third chapter on networking with local professionals—next, in Chapter 4, we'll dig into one of the most potent of all new patient attraction techniques: public speaking.

CHAPTER 4

New Patient Abundance Through Public Speaking

Let's start this chapter with two stories from my personal history as a stage presenter, which I hope will be helpful for you as we begin to explore how to attract new patients with public speaking.

My earliest remembrance of being on stage was when I was in third grade, tackling the daunting assignment of playing the genie in an adaptation of *Aladdin*, being performed in an assembly before the entire student body, the whole faculty, and hundreds of parents.

The plot was simple—students who had talents like dancing or playing the piano rubbed Aladdin's lamp, the genie would appear, and grant them their wish of being a dancer, a flautist, or a pianist, after which they would perform to thunderous applause.

This was very exciting for a seven-year-old, and I worked hard at it until I felt reasonably well-prepared—I knew my lines, had rehearsed my cues, and then, there I was, show time, crouched behind a table on the stage, waiting for the first student to rub the lamp so I could pop up into view.

The curtain went up, and the narrator set the scene. The first kid, the dancer, said her line and started rubbing the lamp. I went to pop up from my hiding spot—and smacked my head on the edge of the table on the way up, knocking myself senseless.

I don't remember a lot about what happened next, except I'm pretty sure I granted the dancer's wish by making her a pianist, after which she went spinning around the stage in a tutu—but it got better from there, and by the time the show was over I was hooked, in spite of my inauspicious entrance.

Now let's fast-forward to the opening of my storefront office in 1980, where I filled my oversized reception area with family, friends, and patients to deliver my first health care class in my new clinic. I had my Renaissance posters clipped to an easel so I could flip them as I spoke, and I enthusiastically launched into my presentation.

"It's seven thirty, and time to begin. Thank you for coming, and welcome to our office." I introduced myself, and as I began my talk, I turned to my charts, lifted the first one... and the clip let loose, scattering them all over the floor.

I bent down, picked up the posters, quickly reorganized them, fastened them better this time, and went on with my talk, which was beautifully received.

I could tell you about all kinds of disasters I weathered as a speaker, from freezing and forgetting my lines to having my fly open, but that would mislead you into thinking it's always so challenging. The truth about being a speaker is that much of what you do is a finely tuned presentation, where the talk goes on essentially as planned, and crazy stuff only happens once in a while.

But I wanted to get it out of the way, for those who have mixed feelings about being a presenter—I thought it would be useful to know that all presenters, yes, all of us, have rough spots we get to break through, emerging on the other side with more experience and more resiliency than before. Stuff happens, and we have to roll with the punches and stay focused on our outcome—to use our presentation to accomplish whatever result we set out to achieve.

We're going to talk a little about what goes into making a quality presentation, and how you can use public speaking to generate an abundance of new patients. But first, let's talk about the purpose of becoming a speaker.

It's often said that the second greatest fear most people suffer is the fear of death, surpassed only by the fear of public speaking—which means that at the funeral, more people would rather be in the box than delivering the eulogy.

But the purpose for becoming a productive and skillful speaker goes far beyond just developing the guts and boldness to stand up there, though of course that helps. If it was only about personal growth, it would be hard for some to get themselves to follow through. But there is a bigger reason to master your stage presentation, and that has to do with making this world a better place with chiropractic.

When you step up to the front of a room, you are taking responsibility to guide those in attendance toward your outcomes—this builds cultural authority. In other words, it positions you, and therefore chiropractic, as something worth hearing about. And that is the main intention of this module—to inspire you to represent chiropractic through group presentation, and become more of a cultural authority to influence more people toward the natural way to health.

Let's start to explore the techniques of presentation so you feel well equipped to put your talk together, a necessary precondition to be an effective speaker.

There are some specialized tools of persuasion that will help you construct the best possible communication, based on people's tendencies to behave consistently with cultural rules and customs. Some of the best research available on this topic is the work of Dr. Robert Cialdini.

Cialdini's Weapons of Influence

In his excellent book *Influence*, Dr. Cialdini discusses six tools he calls the "weapons of influence." There is a cultural hypnosis, or a tendency for people in our society to behave in certain ways in response to certain stimuli, and Cialdini's research identifies these stimuli and how to use them to influence others. This book is certainly worth your reading, and in a nutshell, here are the six tools he explains, and how you can use them in your practice.

Reciprocation means creating a sense of obligation or a need to do something to "even up."

By providing an excellent quality service for someone, and being incredibly nice, courteous, and supportive, you make them feel like they "owe" you something beyond just your fee, so when someone asks if they can do something to reciprocate for your outstanding care and significant impact on their lives, don't deny it—give them a chance to "get even" by referring others they care about. This gives them a win-win-win way of resolving their need to reciprocate.

Commitment and Consistency means asking questions to get small yeses, leading to bigger questions with bigger yeses. For example, you could ask someone, "Is your health important to you?" (They'll say YES.)

"If there were something you could do to be healthier, would you want to know about it?" (They'll say YES.) "If it involved a little time, effort, and money, but the net result was a lifetime of better health, would it be worth it to you to come to a free talk and find out more about it?" (The momentum takes them toward YES.) When people commit and say yes to something, they're more likely to remain consistent by saying yes to related questions, commitment and consistency.

Social Proof means influencing someone based on the opinions of similar others. Tell prospective patients about your successes with people like them, and remind people that those who referred them in did so because they were pleased with the experience. This sets the stage for them to refer others, to add to the social proof of their good decision to come to you.

Liking means getting the person to like you, because it makes it more likely that he or she will respond to you and try not to disappoint you. Just being nice, friendly, loving, and caring goes a long way toward earning people's confidence and increasing their level of compliance. Developing rapport by matching and mirroring also helps.

Authority means applying the leverage of expertise, which is greatly respected in our culture.

By acting authoritative and knowledgeable, and by quoting reputable sources to support your positions, you will be more convincing and sway people toward your way of thinking.

And finally:

Scarcity means the tendency for people to value something that is harder to get or more expensive. This is an argument to maintain the integrity of your fee structure, because people tend to look at free and inexpensive procedures and services as less valuable than more expensive ones.

It should be noted that these tools in and of themselves are not manipulative, but merely persuasive. It's up to the moral character of the person implementing them as to whether they are used honestly or not. Please, always act impeccably—we never "get away" with anything, so use these tools with the highest purpose and integrity only.

Perceived Value, the Ultimate Leverage

Now you have many tools for influencing people and communicating your message. There is another important distinction that will make a significant difference in the quality of your communication.

I wonder if you've ever had any of these experiences:

You talk earnestly to someone you meet at a party about coming in for care, and they seem interested, but they never call.

You give an impassioned report of findings to a new patient, and they don't accept your recommendations, claiming to want a second opinion.

You explain to a patient that you aren't part of their plan, and they never give you a chance to show why you're worth paying extra for.

If you're in practice today, then no doubt you've encountered many situations like these.

You've done your best to get your message across, but many don't respond as you wish they would. In studying doctor-patient communications for the last four decades, I can say with great certainty that there is a unifying factor that makes the big difference in how effective your communication is, and that factor is **perceived value.**

It's an odd concept, perceived value. Isn't there inherent value built into our care that should be obvious to any who look? Why does perception play so large a role?

The willingness to address this issue can be a turning point in your career. Listen to me—we have been trained in our healing art in a very cloistered and discriminating environment, where a special language is spoken, and only club members participate. Most patients and prospective patients have no clue what we're talking about, especially when we launch into technical explanations of our work. This may impress people, but it has no lasting impact other than a good first impression. Soon enough, patients or prospects want to know the answer to one question they are asking themselves—"What's in it for me?"

Now, before you dismiss them as self-serving, you must realize that this is the very same question you had to ask and answer for yourself in deciding to become a chiropractor in the first place. At some point you had to perceive enough value to make you go to school at great expense and inconvenience, set up a practice, also at great expense and inconvenience, and then attempt to create a successful practice, once again, at great expense and inconvenience. The only possible explanation for you going through this ordeal is because you expected that, at some point, you would think it was worth it.

That is exactly what your patients want to feel—that at some point, whatever investment they make of their time, energy and capital, they'll be able to say it was worth it. **Your primary challenge as a chiropractic communicator is to solve the riddle of each individual's formula for perceived value,** and show patients that what you do helps them get something they already want.

Some of you may be thinking, "How can my patient want chiropractic, when he doesn't even know what it is?" This question further illustrates my point. People don't want chiropractic care, they want what they think they will get as a result of chiropractic care. This brings up the concepts of "means" values and "end" values.

You've heard the expression "the end justifies the means." Whether or not you believe this to be true, at least you understand the point—that sometimes you have to go through one set of challenges to resolve another. You could look at it this way; if I asked you, "Why do you work?" you might say, "To make money." But is the reason you work really to obtain small green pictures of dead presidents? Or is it that you can trade those little green slips for other things you really want, like food for your family, new golf clubs, or the ability to support your favorite charity? You see, money in this case is a "means" value, in that it helps you get to an "end" value, such as food, entertainment, or a worthy cause.

The mistake most of us make in communicating to our patients and potential patients is to present our work as an end value, not a means value. This only works if the people were walking around, going, "I really wish I could find someone to correct my subluxations. Do you know anyone like that?" While this is a lovely dream for the future, at this point even the most fervent philosopher would have to admit that only the most advanced thinkers among patients are this evolved.

More often, a patient needs to understand chiropractic care as a means to an end. For that reason, we need to understand what our patient might get out of chiropractic care, either a pleasurable benefit they will enjoy, or a painful consequence they will avoid suffering, or both.

When a patient understands that chiropractic care can keep his spine flexible to extend his golfing career and enhance his score, or can decrease her chances of losing work time from injury, compromising her ability to support her family or advance in her career, or can help a grandfather to be able to play with his grandchildren without pain or danger of harm, the probability of follow-through skyrockets.

It's usually pretty easy to identify your patients' values, since they often state and restate them throughout their conversation with you. They'll say, "Since I hurt myself, I haven't been able to golf," or, "These headaches really interfere with taking proper care of my kids." If the patient or prospect doesn't volunteer such information, you can simply ask, "If you had better health and body function, what would improve in your life?" or, "What does your condition prevent you from doing that you really want to do?"

Questions like these elicit end values, and if not, you can keep asking questions until you get to what you think is really important to the person. The higher the value, the greater the likelihood of compliance.

Your patients need to know what chiropractic can do for them. It's not enough to explain the clinical success rate, since patients expect doctors to think that their work is effective. Your patients need to see how your care helps them improve their lifestyle, avoid limitations and inconveniences, and otherwise restore or enhance something in their lives that is important to them.

That value—the perceived good that manifests or the perceived bad that disappears—is the ultimate leverage in achieving patient compliance. If a patient really understands what's in it for him or her, then you can expect that patient to cooperate, because there is enough perceived value to cause that compliance.

Think about your best, most compliant, most cooperative patients, and notice why they come to you. It's probably because they perceive that your care helps them get something really important to them. The more you help patients perceive the value of your care as it relates to them, the more their level of compliance. It's as simple as that.

The Meaning of your Communication

The point of all this communications material is simply this—the meaning of your communication is the response you get. If a patient or prospect doesn't respond to you in the way you plan, it's not because there's something wrong with them, it's simply that you didn't communicate effectively enough. Take responsibility, learn to accurately assess what kind of person you're dealing with, and you'll dramatically increase the results of your interactions with all people.

Effective Group Presentation—
The Lecture with Something Extra

Now that you've studied effective one-on-one communication, you can begin to extrapolate what you've learned to dealing with groups of people. Becoming skillful at group presentation can dramatically expand your impact on your community and skyrocket your practice. Even if you have little experience so far, you can learn how to be a terrific speaker. Start by identifying the key components to great presenting.

Have you ever seen a speaker mesmerize an audience? Have you ever sat spellbound, taking in every word and marveling at the lecturer's command—the way the listeners responded, the pure power and potency of the presentation? If you're like me, you really appreciate a terrific stage performance, and the purpose of this section is to create a model of an excellent public speaker and to show you how to apply it to attract new patients every day.

The Five Components of Great Speaking

There are five components to a great speaker, five areas that can be refined and mastered so that the presenter can be as effective as possible. By learning how to balance and blend these five components, you can improve the quality of your presentations.

Friendliness and Fun

The first component I call friendliness and fun, and the reason I begin here is because if you don't get your audience to like you, then they won't be able to get past that to receive your message. So, the first thing you have to pay attention to is to be likeable, to enjoy yourself and to help the listeners enjoy themselves. Remember that Cialdini talked about liking and being likeable as being an important tool of influence. So, whatever you can do to get your audience to like you will make it more likely that they will listen and be persuaded by what you say.

The basics are obvious enough. Smile, and open with pleasing gestures and tonalities. You want to get rapport with the audience; in other words, you want to create a bond, a feeling of comfort and connection between you and your listeners. (Review the sections on rapport in Chapters 2 and 3 or read the section on rapport in the book *Unlimited Power* by Anthony Robbins.)

In this context, when you get out on stage, look around and notice the tone in the room. The composite energy of the room will help you decide your opening pace. If the room seems lively and fast-paced, then begin your talk with a quick pace. If the room is more mellow, then start with a mellower pace and tonality.

Matching your approach to the audience is a powerful tool for creating rapport, and once you have a good connection, you can start to shift the energy in whatever direction suits your presentation. Light and entertaining ... authoritative and didactic ... motivating and enthusiastic ... whatever mood you want to create, you have to have a connection with the audience first so they'll like you enough to follow along. Whether you call it charisma, animal magnetism, likability or whatever, getting your audience to accept you and feel comfortable makes it more likely that people will enjoy and respond to your presentation.

Congruency and Physiology

The second components of being a great speaker are called congruency and physiology. These are terms that are used in neurolinguistic programming and they can be defined as follows:

Congruency means showing no inner and outer conflict. In other words, the speaker comes across as honest, sincere, and truly meaning and believing what he or she is saying. This is very important in a speaker because whether it's fair or not, an audience has to buy the messenger before it will buy the message.

So, how can you come across as believable? That's where the second term, physiology, comes in. The word *physiology* in this context means what you are doing with your body. This is important because some physiologies are perceived as congruent and some are perceived as incongruent. Your challenge is to select physiologies that are perceived as congruent.

Here are some pointers. First, be yourself. Authenticity is hard to fake. As you get more skillful as a speaker, your stage persona will become more flexible and you'll have a wider range of "yous" to choose from. For now, you should just concentrate on being honest and sincere and use the posture, facial expressions, gestures, and tonality that go along with that. You may want to practice in front of a mirror or even shoot a video so you can check yourself. Do you seem believable to you? If so, you are probably on track. If not, then here are a few things you can work on.

Is your appearance appropriate? Make sure your clothing is properly arranged to avoid distracting people. Check your posture. Symmetry is very important in conveying congruency. Your weight should be divided evenly over both legs, and your movements should be balanced, even bilateral, if possible—outstretched arms, clasped hands, full-faced smile, etc.

If you're going to use asymmetry, use it purposefully, like a specific gesture—for example, a salute or fist, a sideways glance for humorous effect, or a wink. Avoid accidental asymmetries like an off-centered gaze, or a nervous or misplaced smile that might confuse or distort your message. Flirtatious glances or shifty-eyed looks are notorious for causing distrust, and inconsistencies in tonality are also telltale. Practice your craft so your facial expressions, timing, and tone of voice match up well with the message you are putting across.

Also, keep your attention focused outward on the audience. They'll need to feel you are paying attention to them, rather than making it seem that you are thinking about what you are saying. That feeling of spontaneity adds to your congruency, and when your audience perceives you as congruent, they trust you, because they feel that you really believe in what you're saying.

Skill, Precision, and Preparation

Now that the audience likes you and trusts you, it's time for the third component of a great speaker—skill, precision, and preparation. If you're going to be an outstanding public speaker, then you have to know what you're going to say and then, say it well.

Depending on your style and experience, you may want to write out your entire script, or you may prefer to work from an outline. Plan your presentation so that it has an opening, a body, and a closing.

Think of your talk like a show. Ease the audience in, get them involved, tell them what you need to tell them, and when you're finished, leave them different and better than when they arrived. The content of your talk should be more than just accurate, it should be structured so that the key points are stated several different times in several different ways because the repetition will help the listeners learn.

Rehearse your talk and use mirrors, tape recorders, videos, or dry runs in front of friends or supporters. The more you practice, the more distinctions you'll be able to make, and this refinement process will increase your skill and precision. Work on your delivery and your timing so that when lecture day comes, you'll feel prepared.

Creativity

Once you know how to get the group to like you and trust you, and you've prepared well, you're in position to add the fourth component of great speaking, and that is creativity. This is where you begin to bring your presentation alive, to make it unique, to give it personality—in short, to make it you.

Are you tastefully funny? Work it into your presentation. Do you have a very expressive face or voice? Use it to your advantage. Are you artistically inclined? Design your own PowerPoints, charts, overheads, and handouts. Think of innovative ways to deliver your material. A creative approach will help your audience learn better and remember you as someone who had something valuable and interesting to offer. Try using stories or metaphors to convey your concepts, and you'll keep the group's attention better.

For example, some of you have probably used the iceberg metaphor—that the person's symptoms are just the tip of the iceberg, with the cause being much bigger and below the surface. Or, perhaps you've talked about the garden hose, or dimmed a bulb with a rheostat to demonstrate a subluxation. These may seem a bit corny, but like all clichés, they persist because they still work.

Your challenge is to come up with novel ways to get your point across. Try lots of different stuff to find out what works for you and when. Experiment with video or a live demonstration of some sort. Use miraculous or emotional case histories for impact. Design a slide presentation around your personal approach. Get several sets of charts, and mix and match for variety. Play Whitney Houston's "Greatest Love of All" or Michael Jackson's "Heal The World" behind your closing. Use the Chiropractic Clipping Service to collect articles, photos, and graphs that support your material, and transfer them to PowerPoint slides.

You want to appeal to all of the senses. Give the audience plenty to look at, listen to, and feel, and you'll be using the fourth component, creativity.

At this point, you know how to get an audience to like you and trust you. You have prepared a great talk, rehearsed it, and added creative touches to make it interesting and memorable.

These steps alone will make you a very competent and entertaining lecturer. There is another level though, and in order to achieve it ... in order to create the lecture with something extra, you need to use the fifth component of great presentation, and that is—passion!

Passion

Your level of excitement and enthusiasm is the power that drives your talk beyond information to communication. When your energy and commitment come out in your performance, your audience is swept up in the moment and compelled to participate. Remember how important what you're doing really is. When you teach people about chiropractic, you could be saving their lives, or sparing their children needless suffering, or providing relief for someone who has hurt for so long. It's so special what we do as chiropractors, so don't be afraid to tell people passionately. Make sure to close your presentation with as much emotion as possible.

For example, a story or favorite case history works well as a passionate closing. Throughout most of your talk you had them looking and listening, but at the end, when they get to decide how what you've told them about really affects them in their lives, you want them to feel. A wonderful speaker and sports commentator, legendary basketball coach Jim Valvano, was asked what his formula was for creating a successful talk. He said, "I just try to do three things—make them laugh, make them think, and make them cry." If you keep that in mind, then before too long you'll be delivering the lecture with something extra.

Now that we have a handle on how to compose an effective presentation, let's direct our attention toward using these tools to attract large numbers of new patients.

New Patient Abundance Through Public Speaking

With so many promotional ideas, like screenings, health fairs, patient appreciation days, advertising, social media marketing, and charity events, the granddaddy of all new patient strategies is the patient lecture. Since the beginning, people have been learning about chiropractic by sitting and listening to someone talk about how our unique approach can help them to be healthier.

The purpose of this section is to give you a strategy for taking this excellent tool and expanding its impact, because there are many people in your community who are not yet aware of what chiropractic can do for them, but would be very receptive to the message. In order to get to these people, there are some specific action steps you can take that will fill your lecture schedule with productive, meaningful speaking engagements.

Before you're ready to start this marketing process, though, there are some specific preliminary steps that you must take in order to be prepared when these speaking opportunities arise.

The first and most obvious point is—have something to say! This may seem silly, because after all, you are an expert on a variety of related topics. With a little preparation, you can present quite a bit of material that will be both useful and interesting for just about any audience. The key here is to take the time to prepare so that whatever advantage you can get, you can take.

There are three aspects to preparing for your talk: researching the needs of your audience, compiling the appropriate material, and sculpting the material into a finished presentation that is relevant and useful for this particular audience.

Who is your Audience?

Start by thinking about potential target audiences. Who are you going to be speaking to? A general audience? Businesspeople? Young families? Seniors? The flavor and tone of your lecture will vary tremendously based on the group you are addressing, so before you compile the material for your talk, consider the interests, needs, and values of your target audience. For example, seniors might be more interested in a class on slowing the aging process than one on sports injury, where a younger audience might relate better to sports. Carefully research the needs of your prospects—the closer you get to making them feel that you are speaking directly to them, the more likely they will respond to your message and take the action you want—to become your patient.

When you book the lecture, find out from whomever you are dealing with about the audience. What is the age range? What are some of the common interests and values? What related topics have they already heard about and enjoyed in previous talks? The more you understand their needs, the better you can custom-tailor the presentation and the better you can expect your results to be.

Design A Great Talk

Once you know what the group wants and expects, you can compile the subject matter of the talk. There is so much material that can be presented; you'll need to focus on relevant aspects to keep your lecture to the desired length. Create a filing system for your lecture materials, and develop a repertoire of different topics you can address for different audiences.

By establishing a basic format to your talk, you can mix and match different information, stories, anecdotes, illustrations, and examples that apply specifically to the group you want to address. For instance, there are certain remarks that will be part of pretty much any talk you prepare—comments that introduce you and qualify you as an authority, basic information about chiropractic and the impact it has on people's health, and a powerful, persuasive closing. But, how about all the stuff in between?

That's your opportunity to show the group that you have something to offer them that specifically fills some need, solves some problem, or addresses some issue that helps them in an obvious and tangible way. For example, sport enthusiasts of all kinds will relate to the positive comments superstars like Joe Montana, Jerry Rice, or Michael Jordan have made about chiropractic's role in their health routine, so scare up an article or video to this effect and quote it liberally in talks to health clubs, gyms, sports hobbyist groups, or teenagers.

Or, if addressing seniors, who may or may not care as much about Jerry Rice, you can concentrate more on the positive impact chiropractic care has on keeping the spine mobile and flexible, decreasing the likelihood of degenerative disease restricting their ability to get around.

Or, if you're talking to blue-collar workers, focus more on family values, and how chiropractic can get them back on the job faster after an injury so their livelihood is not threatened. You may also want to use the "Discover Wellness Presents" lecture series to promote wellness in your community.

Are you getting the idea here? Once you identify the audience's needs, include support material that shows them how what you do helps them get something they want.

Become a Professional Presenter

Once you've compiled the material that applies to the group you are preparing for, polish the presentation in rehearsal. If you are using visual aids, practice integrating them into the talk. Remember my story about the charts that came loose from the easel—a little better planning and rehearsal could have avoided that embarrassment and inconvenience.

This type of rehearsal gives you a chance to work out any rough spots in your talk. When I'm developing a talk I often use a mirror, a flip cam or tape recorder, and a stopwatch.

By rehearsing in front of a mirror, you can be sure that you are presenting the proper image. Match your movements, gestures, and facial expressions to the subject matter, and avoid anything distracting or inappropriate.

Tape or video your rehearsals so you can watch or listen back and check tonality, cadence, and timing, and listen to the entire tape at least once to make sure the whole talk works as a package. Don't be surprised by the sound of your voice on tape—everyone feels that way in the beginning. If there are any stories or illustrations that don't seem to work, fix or replace them—better to make your corrections in rehearsal, so by the time you present your talk it is polished and professional.

Find out in advance how long you will have to speak, and time your rehearsals so you finish at the right time. Once you get some experience under your belt, you'll develop an inner clock that keeps you on time, but while you're learning to do this, work with a stopwatch. Make sure no section of your talk seems too long, and plan to leave enough time for a proper closing.

Now that you've done your homework, it's show time! How can we turn this lecture approach into lots of new patients?

In-Office Lectures

There are two broad categories of lecture opportunities—in-office lectures, and out-of-office lectures. In-office lectures can be either basic, new patient orientation-type lectures or more advanced, regular patient-type lectures. Make the new patient orientation part of all new patients' basic training by telling them in the report of findings that all patients in your office attend this lecture, and the result is that your patients get well faster and understand how to help themselves better.

Or if you prefer a softer approach, say that you offer the class because most patients have the same basic questions about your program of care, and your presentation is based on the answers to those questions.

Encourage them to bring their spouses and/or any friends who might be interested in health, or those who might have a problem and want to find out if chiropractic can help them. You can set it up as a workshop, and tell the patients that they should bring a partner to work with. You can have them check each other's hips, shoulders, and head tilt, and everyone has a good time and learns something. You can say, "Because this is an interactive workshop, please bring a partner to work with, or one will be assigned to you." Since people would typically prefer to work with someone they know, this increases the likelihood that they will bring a guest.

Advanced classes should be geared toward perceived need—you can teach classes on advanced chiropractic philosophy, brain-based wellness, stress reduction, nutrition, safe exercising, yoga, or even choose a "condition of the month" if you like. Giving patients the opportunity to learn and bring friends and family to learn results in not only more new patients, but also better new patients who begin care informed, enthusiastic, and willing to cooperate. Put up a sign-in sheet that announces the topic, date, and time of the class, and encourage people to attend and bring people.

We'll talk about health care class in more detail, but first let's direct our attention toward outside lectures.

Outside Lectures

Outside lectures require a little more planning, but are still easy to set up. Decide who you would like to speak to. Businesses, service organizations, hobby clubs, religious institutions, health clubs, schools, support groups, seniors' homes, civic or special interest groups—there are many potential audiences to choose from. Decide who will be interested in and respond to your message, and use this strategy to contact them.

Call them to find out who is in charge of special programs, and get a name and address to send some information. Compose a letter that explains the benefits of your presentations and send it to the appropriate person.

A week later, call the person and set up a meeting to further discuss the details. By the time you meet the person, you'll have had three or four contacts, which substantially increases the probability of getting the speaking engagement.

In the meeting, ask lots of questions. "Tell me about your company. What are your needs? What are some problems that have been causing you stress or costing you money? What health information would be valuable to your people? Are there any health concerns you may have?" Conduct the interview to expose the benefits that will be gained as a result of your talk, and the consequences that will be suffered without it. Offer choices of different topics so the individual can choose one that is suitable.

When you are closing the interview, your goal is to make a date for a speaking engagement, so steer the conversation that way with yes questions—for example, you can say, "Now that we've talked about the content of these talks, can you see how it would be beneficial to your group to get this information?" Or, "You see how not knowing about this valuable material could cost you money, don't you?" Or, "If providing this talk for your membership saved them needless suffering and helped them be healthier and more productive, you'd want that, wouldn't you?"

These types of closing questions will increase your batting average at booking these talks—you won't get everyone to say yes, but plan to contact enough prospects to generate the number of talks you want to do, depending on your new patient goals. I have certainly heard of doctors signing up forty and fifty new patients from a single lecture, though even getting two or three makes it worth your while. If you do two lectures a month and get two new patients from each lecture, which would be fifty additional new patients per year, that would generate an additional hundred or hundred fifty office visits a month or more, and probably $100-150K more in collections over the year—and that's on a modest estimate. Many doctors average five or ten new patients per talk. You can do the math!

Public speaking is one of the very best ways to keep new patients flowing into your office. It costs very little money, positions you as an authority, creates a presence in your community, and is among the most productive techniques you can use to create new patient abundance in your office. Set up the system as described here, develop yourself into an outstanding presenter, and discover how you can talk your way to a more successful practice.

Health Care Class

Now, let's direct our attention toward health care class, one of the most powerful and productive patient engagement techniques. Whether you provide your health talk in the office only or take it on the road, it's a great tool for both educating patients and attracting new lives to serve.

Your health care class not only helps others understand the scope of your services to create more value for your care, it also gives more people the chance to discover who you are, what you do, and how it benefits them, giving you the opportunity to attract more new patients.

The first step in this process is to simply make the decision and commit to doing a regular health care class, also known as a special consultation, lay lecture, or wellness orientation workshop. The reason for this commitment is because it's easy to give yourself excuses as to why you should not give your HCC on a given day or evening... you know, people don't want to show up, you don't have enough new patients, the CA doesn't want to stay, and so on.

Making this commitment usually leads to greater success, not only because of the obvious benefit of presenting information, but also because speaking consistently rapidly improves your skill, giving you even greater results as you continue to grow.

Health care class can be offered any day or evening that you feel is in the best interest of your patients and you. Many chiropractors choose a day or evening that is not a full day of office hours, but this is entirely up to you. The best frequency seems to be either every week or every other week—I think it's better to do them each week.

The first question most doctors ask when they plan to start doing a regular health care class is, "How do I get people there?" Usually, you'll get the best attendance if the doctor requests the patient's participation. The time to introduce patients to the concept is at the report of findings. This is when the patient is most engaged and most likely to do the things you ask them to do because this is when most patients are excited to start their care and are compelled to follow through on your guidance.

After you have given your recommendations, you can use this sample dialogue to attract more patients into your health care class.

"Lastly, Mr. Patient, we have a special consultation on Tuesday evenings at 7:30 PM... All new patients are requested to attend. The reason we ask all new patients to participate is because we have found from experience that when patients come to this presentation, they get the best possible results in the shortest period of time, at the least amount of cost! Do you want that?"

Of course, most people will reply yes to this question simply because saying no is not a viable option. Once you get confirmation from the patient that it IS in their best interest to attend your special consultation, you can then ask the following question: "We suggest that you bring your spouse or significant other, or maybe a friend or other family member. Since part of the consultation is also a workshop, you can choose to bring a partner with you, or someone will be assigned to you. Which would you prefer?"

Most people would prefer to work with someone they know. Very few people feel comfortable enough to work with a stranger, so this invites more new people, both to support their friends or significant others, or for them to become patients when they hear the chiropractic story so they can apply health and wellness reasoning to their own lives.

Sometimes patients may have a legitimate reason why they cannot attend the special consultation. While it is never recommended to become argumentative with a patient, the following alternative is offered, which can increase your chances of their attendance either now, or in the future.

If a patient says, "Doc, I just can't make it that night," the DC can say, "I can appreciate how busy you must be—I just want you to know that from my experience, when a patient does not attend this health talk for whatever reason, sometimes they don't respond as quickly, don't get quite the same results. They may even end up spending a bit more money... are you okay with that?"

The vast majority of people will not be okay with that and will usually ask the following question, "When's the next one?" While we certainly can set a goal for a 100% attendance, a good goal could be to have 85-90% compliance, with guest attendance at 50% or better.

Once you begin instituting the health care class into your normal and regular routine, you will find that patients will, in fact, get better results, stay longer, and make your practice more fulfilling and enjoyable while becoming more profitable as well.

Make it your Policy

As backup to this procedure, it's a good idea to include this passage in your office policy statement, to be read and signed by each new patient.

The purpose of requiring all new patients to attend a Special Consultation or Wellness Orientation Workshop is to help you learn about your body, especially the brain, spine, and nerve system. Since chiropractic is not like the practice of medicine, and is probably new to you, please let us explain to you how to help us help you get well faster. We have found that patients who have attended seem to respond better, because they understand the cause of their problem and what we are attempting to do to correct it.

In a proper doctor-patient relationship, both the doctor and the patient have various responsibilities if you are to receive maximum benefits in the minimum amount of time. Natural healing requires cooperation!

Your attendance at the Special Consultation is essential! It is part of your program of care. Further, we invite you to bring your spouse or another family member, so he or she can understand too, and learn to assist you in your quest to regain your health.

Friends and relatives may also attend, as this is a terrific way for them to find out the value and benefits of chiropractic care and how it suits their needs. Just ask at the front desk to reserve a place for your guests.

A quick note to new presenters who may experience a little stage fright—public speaking does take some guts, but you'll be amazed how quickly you get comfortable doing it. Just think about it—you can give a report of findings to a patient, and you can give the report of findings to both the patient and the spouse, you've done it before. That's an example of speaking in front of two people. Can you do this with one more person in the room? How about two? You get my point—you can do this…and you'll be glad you did. Get strong, practice enough so you can be confident, and get started.

Make your Health Care Class a Personal Statement

Now that you have a patient and his or her guest coming to your special consultation, you may be asking yourself, "What do I talk about?" This is the easiest part of doing a health care class, since the information you are about to provide is a reflection of the purpose and philosophy that you have—both personally and professionally.

There are so many benefits, so much information and knowledge that you can impart unto your patients, and by doing so in a group setting you save time, thereby increasing your capacity to grow your practice.

Some DCs choose to use a PowerPoint presentation in their office, while others simply use a white board or charts… still others use nothing at all and simply engage their patients in a philosophical discussion. What you speak about in your health care class is not most important! What is important is the energy, attitude, and enthusiasm you bring to the subject matter you're speaking about.

Ask yourself, "Why did I become a chiropractor? What does my ideal practice really look like? Does doing this class take me closer or further away from my ideal practice?" The goal is to help patients more clearly understand what you are doing to help them!

Your opening should qualify you as an expert without being pompous. Using an anecdote from your practice or an opening metaphor or story welcomes people into your presentation. The body of the talk is a unique reflection of your practice philosophy.

Therefore, no two HCCs are the same. Write a class that features your perspective on health and wellness, and in addition to telling the chiropractic story, you can include information about exercise, nutrition, sleeping habits, a positive mental attitude, posture, or anything else you believe should be emphasized. This is why this is such a powerful tool!

Most chiropractic offices work at correcting subluxations, so introducing some concepts of chiropractic philosophy may be called for. You can share these four basic ideas, which I first heard promoted this way from Drs. Patrick Gentempo and Christopher Kent.

Four Basic Concepts

1. The body is a self-healing and self-regulating organism.

2. The nerve system is the master control system of the body.

3. Anything that interferes with nerve control, like a subluxation, is bad.

4. Anything that corrects or reduces nerve interference, like an adjustment, is good.

Make it a Workshop

Earlier in this book, it was mentioned that the patient should be bringing in a partner for the "workshop" portion of the special consultation. The workshop is an opportunity to get people out of the chairs and get their bodies moving so they can more fully pay attention to the information you are sharing.

The idea is to "train" the participants to examine the spine from behind by comparing hip height, shoulder height, and head position. Ask patients to get with their partners, and pair up any who have no partners, to begin the workshop.

Using the "I" Test

To introduce this interactive part of the class, I used to announce, "Now we're going to do an 'I' test." When people looked at me funny, I explained, "It's not an eye test (pointing at my eye) it's an 'I' test, like the letter I. You know how a capital I has a straight line up and down, and a short line across the top and bottom? Your spine, shoulders, and hips should look like that, and we're all going to examine each other to see who passes the 'I' test." Participants always got the joke, and it lightens the mood, since people often don't feel that comfortable looking at each other and touching each other.

Have one of the patients act as the "doctor" and the other act as the "patient." Have the patient stand with their back to the doctor and have the doctor do a postural screening while you are informing them about what to look for. They will see people with all different types of postural distortions... high shoulder on the left, head tilted toward the right, and so on. Then, you can point out how these small postural distortions can put pressure on other areas of the spine and nervous system, which is part of the training you have as a chiropractor!

Now you can explain how distortion and the nerve interference that results from it can rob the body of the ability for all the other factors to contribute to good health. Your patients will begin to understand how this information fits together, which will give them the best opportunity to live a healthier lifestyle.

Now that your patients are more fully aware of the benefits you provide with your adjustments and other forms of care in your office, it's time to give others the opportunity to be helped by you as well. This is why your closing of the talk is so important. It invites patients to renew their commitment, and gives prospective patients the chance to register their desire for a healthier lifestyle.

Learn to Close Effectively

Here's one example of the many ways you can close your talk.

"I do these classes for two reasons...the first is to provide my patients with the information about what chiropractic is and is not, and I believe we have accomplished that this evening...would you all agree?" You'll usually get some applause or acknowledgment for sharing what you know. "The second reason I do these is to provide our guests an opportunity to find out how chiropractic can help them, too!

"And, in all my years of experience, I have never been able to accomplish that goal without your participation, by simply having a checkup. Now, I have no idea if you need care or not, but I can tell you this—if you haven't had a checkup, you probably could benefit from one, either to catch a problem early, or to get the peace of mind of knowing everything is fine.

"So I'm not saying you need care or don't need care, I don't know that yet. What am I offering here?"

The patients will reply: "A checkup!"

The DC then says, "So what do you think you should do?"

The patients almost invariably say: "I think I want to schedule a checkup!"

You will find that the patients will be more cooperative if you ask questions and allow them to make the decision, rather than making your class "mandatory" or being too assertive or heavy-handed when suggesting a checkup or examination. Most chiropractors report that this Socratic methodology is gentle and respectful, yet works well and helps to maximize their results.

I don't recommend a "free" examination when presenting your invitational offer during your health care class. You may risk sending the wrong message to the patient. Do you value a free service the way you value something you pay for? It might feel good for a moment, but do you value it? So, while many chiropractors offer some form of a discounted fee, it is better to keep your usual and customary fee for an examination when scheduling the checkup. If you vary from this at all, you must check your local, state, and federal regulations to be sure you are in compliance.

Some chiropractors offer a consultation at no charge to any patient who wants to see if there's a good fit, and if you offer this service as part of your regular office policy, it fits nicely into your closing. It isn't recommended to offer free services as an inducement to begin care, but if you offer a complimentary consultation as part of your policy, then that's a suitable invitation to a prospective patient to gather enough information to decide whether or not your services are a good fit for his or her needs.

Once you establish good systems and execution for your regular health care class, you can expand your speaking schedule to include advanced in-office lectures.

Advanced Health Care Class

Advanced classes should be geared toward perceived need—as I mentioned before, you can teach classes on advanced chiropractic philosophy, brain-based wellness, stress reduction, nutrition, safe exercising, or a health topic like a "condition of the month," if you like.

Sharing these distinctions results in a better informed and more compliant patient, because they comprehend why they are coming and their role in the process. For that reason be proactive, and direct your evolving patients into your advanced health care class track—they'll all benefit, and some may even decide to become chiropractors. So, take it seriously and get people enrolled.

Remember that the focus of this module is to bring in new patients every day, and skillful presenters can do so just with speaking—between health care class, advanced health care class, and outside lectures, you will be able to figure out how many talks you need to do to attract the number of new patients you desire. If you work sixteen days a month, and you want to attract sixteen new patients, one each day, then you need to know how efficiently you attract people through speaking.

If you typically start one new patient from each health care class, and you do one health care class each week, that should bring in four new patients each month. If your outside talks average about three new patients each, then to get to sixteen, you'd need to do one outside talk each week. Of course this is if you expect to use only speaking as your only new patient attraction strategy. I just want you to see that it is quite possible to choose any of these techniques and get new patients every day by using them effectively.

Public speaking is one of the most powerful new patient attraction techniques you can apply. With a little planning and a little experience, you too can be standing at the front of the room, guiding people toward a better quality of life, and building the practice you really want while earning more money and making the world a better place, too.

Points to Remember

1. According to Cialdini, there are six basic tools you can use to influence people—reciprocation, commitment and consistency, social proof, liking, authority, and scarcity.

2. There are five elements to a great presentation—friendliness and fun, congruency and physiology, preparation and skill, creativity, and passion.

3. Whether you plan inside or outside lectures, basic or advanced health care classes, you must close effectively to get the best results possible.

Actions to Take

1. Develop a model of a great, all-purpose closing that you can adapt to a variety of different talks.

2. Decide how often you'd like to speak, based on how many patients you typically attract from a talk, and begin to create a plan to arrange for those talks.

Questions to Ponder

1. What do you look for in a speaker that impresses you?

2. What kind of audience do you feel responds best to you at this time, and how could you expand your influence to reach more people?

You should now have a good working knowledge of how to offer a persuasive presentation from the stage—now, in Chapter 5, let's discuss how to design and implement effective promotions, both inside your office and in your community.

CHAPTER 5
Promotions and Five-by-Five Marketing

When I first got out of chiropractic college, I felt like I had the flame of life in my hands. I just knew that whatever community I settled in, people were going to flock to see me in droves.

So wasn't I surprised when I hung my shingle and made myself available to see patients, that at first not much was going on. My first patient was referred by my wife, Regina. Her friend, Suzy, who was a physical therapist, was my first chiropractic miracle case while I was still a student. She was Patient #001.

My second patient was a woman named Gail, who was the best friend of Dr. Bob Hoffman's mom, Bev, may she rest in peace. Gail brought in her sons, who went on to become chiropractors—then Bob's mom came in, with his brothers, who also went on to become chiropractors—Bob was still in school, and I have never forgotten his trust and respect in sending me his loved ones to take care of.

But before long, Bob ran out of friends and family to refer, and I realized that if I wanted a busy practice, I was going to have to go out and find some new patients.

I saw some flyers around town advertising a health fair, and I took down the contact number and called to see if I could participate in some way. I really wanted to speak, but they were only planning on setting up tables arranged in rows, so I took one of those tables. I think I paid a hundred bucks to be one of about fifty local health professionals exhibiting in a parking lot of a neighborhood shopping mall. It was the summer of 1978. I'd been in practice for about three months, and I was about to turn twenty-five years old.

In anticipation, I prepared the best I could, trying to make up for my inexperience with enthusiasm. I wrote and printed a one-page manifesto about chiropractic, hand-stamped some chiropractic patient literature with my name, address, and phone number, made sure I had plenty of cards, and when the day arrived, I grabbed my trusty model spine and headed over to the fair.

This was before the days of the NeuroInfiniti and the Insight—in fact, at the time, a plumb line was considered high tech, and I didn't even have one of those—just the flame of life in my hands. But I still felt well equipped, and excited about the event.

I thought there were going to be crowds of people there, as the sponsors of the event had promised, but when they started admitting participants, there were about a dozen people, wandering from booth to booth to satisfy their curiosity.

And you know, it didn't get a lot better from there. There were never more than about twenty people there, lost in this tangle of rows of booths spread over this large parking lot. I kept a good attitude, trying to talk to people who walked by, but I wasn't very skillful, and they were already overwhelmed by the other doctors and vendors they had spoken to.

It looked like it was going to be a wash, and I was contemplating cleaning up and heading out early, when a youngish man approached me and asked if I was the new chiropractor across the street from Queens General Hospital, and I said yes. He said he had heard some good things about me, and wanted to come in for a checkup.

Well, that patient stayed with me for years and sent me about twenty-five referrals. If I had left that health fair ten minutes earlier, it would have cost me about fifty thousand dollars, not to mention the opportunity to help dozens of people.

Fast-forward about six and a half years, when I was practicing in my home office in Syosset, New York. Every year I bought a giant five-foot Christmas stocking filled with games, toys, and candy, and did a drawing that people could enter by bringing a new unwrapped Christmas gift I could donate to a local charity. I still remember the excitement and joy on the part of the winner that year, whose family had to spread their limited resources over five children—they all had a very Merry Christmas that year.

The point is, there are many ways to promote your chiropractic practice, but the best promotions not only bring in new people for you to serve, they also do as much good as possible. When you keep that in mind, your promotions will be that much more successful.

Many chiropractors resist promoting their practices, feeling that it's difficult, inconvenient, and messy, and at times that's true. But the end product... you know, it's kind of like changing a diaper. You have a completely different experience if you pay attention to *who's* in the diaper, instead of *what's* in the diaper.

The Event Driven Practice

One of the most successful chiropractic promotional systems of all time is The Event Driven Practice, developed by Dr. Bob Hoffman, co-founder of The Masters Circle (with Dr. Larry Markson and myself.)

The Event Driven Practice is a concept of practice promotion that recommends planning a marketing calendar of compelling and relevant events that engage patients at a deeper level, and expose more people to the miraculous healing benefits of chiropractic care.

Developing an event-driven practice is an insider secret that successful practitioners use to attract and build relationships with more ideal patients.

You can use these ideas to develop a simple and highly personalized turnkey system to move forward and bring your practice to a higher level.

When you follow The Event Driven Practice procedures, your marketing calendar is more likely to stimulate you to take consistent and persistent action. You'll find yourself concentrating your new patient energy into high productivity strategies. You'll empower your marketing, spread the word about your work, position yourself as a leader in your community, and have fun creating the practice of your dreams.

It's fun and productive to create invitations, flyers, letters, and press releases, customized for your practice and used to publicize your events. In fact, The Event Driven Practice products actually offer many variations of these set-up materials, some of which we'll be going over in this chapter.

The concept is to plan an event between one and four times each month, depending on the complexity and scope of the project. Some are simple and inexpensive, or even free, like Hug Day or International Smile Week.

Others are elaborate and require more financial resources, like a Patient Appreciation Dinner or a Movie Night.

Finding the right balance for your practice will allow you to have a well-rounded marketing calendar that consistently produces results.

You'll need to assemble your action plan, considering lead time, scripting, preparation and follow up, to ensure the most effective and efficient results. It takes the guesswork out of turning your practice into a new patient machine. You'll get some examples of these concepts and materials as we go forward.

The Event Driven Practice solves the chiropractor's age-old problem—attracting, retaining, and recalling patients. It helps you to educate your community on health, wellness, and safety. It raises your vibration and attractiveness by increasing the energy field surrounding you, which draws patients into your practice.

The Event Driven Practice is not only about bringing new patients through the door, but also about keeping the patients you currently have, as well as recalling the ones whom you haven't seen in a while.

Relationship building is the common thread to accomplishing these goals. It's how you can establish yourself as an expert in your field, and show the community what makes you and your practice unique, thereby retaining, recalling, and attracting patients into your practice.

Traditionally, any sales process was based on some kind of seduction. Luring people into a sale with shiny objects, broad promises, and smarmy enthusiasm was prevalent in the marketplace. But as the health care consumer becomes more savvy, seductive approaches wane in popularity and effectiveness. Patients tend to pursue quality relationships with their product and service providers instead of quick fixes.

That transition is still underway, but there is a growing need for doctors to bring people toward them by applying the law of attraction.

That's why events such as patient appreciation dinners, workshops or lectures in schools, businesses, and organizations, health care class, themed events, and networking with other professionals are more apt to bring in your ideal patients. These days, it works better to attract patients than to attempt to seduce them with a slick line or a bargain price.

The wave of the future in health care is the Wellness Revolution! More than ever before the general public is open-minded to a natural and holistic approach to health, and many are ready to try new things. The time is perfect for your sane and sensible wellness approach, especially a brain-based wellness approach.

At its best, an event-driven practice becomes a special place to go, with a reputation for sponsoring exciting, informative, and worthwhile promotions that everyone benefits from. The sky is the limit—there's no shortage of people out there, and they can all, to varying degrees, benefit from your services. You've got to find a way to engage them so they can choose to follow you to a better quality of life.

Before we dig into the specifics of generating large numbers of new patients with your promotions, let's look at some important distinctions Dr. Hoffman makes about how to turn your marketing into relationship building.

Relationship Building: The Four Rs

To many chiropractors, the word *marketing* feels somehow unsavory—but relationship building sounds appealing.

In the modern chiropractic world, effective marketing is based on building relationships with people in your community.

Here are the four *R*s of building relationships with your patients and your community:

Relate: Make the Connection

The first *R* of relationship building is to Relate, to make a connection, to generate rapport. When people meet and get a sense of comfort around each other, it begins a bond that feels good and allows positive movement.

Find commonalities between you and the people you meet to build rapport. Ask questions to better understand people—pay attention to their needs and wants, and relate to them. And, of course, match and mirror to engage at the physiological level.

Choose to be optimistic—the success of your relationship begins with aligning with the other and exemplifying the qualities they'd want in a relationship.

Reassure: Have a Friend on the Inside

The second *R* of relationship building is to Reassure, to give someone the feeling that they have a friend on the inside.

Rapport begins when commonalities are discovered and acknowledged. Next, you move the relationship forward by reassuring your new relationship mate that you have something to offer, that you're willing to be there for them, so they start to develop trust and belief, to value the relationship and see what could be in it for them.

Listen actively so they are encouraged to open up to you. Show them you are engaged with a nod of the head and a smile, or by paraphrasing what was said back to them so they see that you consider what they are saying is important.

When you follow these simple patterns, the person will tend to feel that you truly understand them, and when people feel they are being listened to, they are much more likely to want to perpetuate and enhance the relationship.

Reinforce: Cement the Bond

The third *R* is to Reinforce, to cement the bond between you. This occurs naturally when people know more about each other and feel more comfortable with each other, and that's when communication is optimized.

You'll feel compelled to support the other's observations or build on their arguments.

We've spoken at length about matching and mirroring, and of course this cannot be overlooked as an advantage in generating the most profound connection with people. Again, it demonstrates that people who are like each other tend to like each other, and becomes more and more natural as the relationship unfolds.

Once rapport is established, it gets easier to see things from the other person's perspective, to understand how he or she feels and to work toward making the relationship satisfying for both parties.

React: Work the Relationship

The fourth R is to React, to work the relationship, to take the actions within the context of your engagement that move the relationship forward, improving the quality of life for all concerned.

As you study human behavior and get to know how people will tend to act, you can use your observations and distinctions to become an expert at relationship building. There's nowhere to invest your time, energy, and resources that will yield a better return.

It's your responsibility to create new relationships and improve old ones. You will discover this to be a foundational stone in promoting your office, whether you are developing new relationships with prospective patients or inter-referral resources, or enhancing relationships with patients and strategic partners you've worked effectively with for years.

Practice these relationship-building techniques to increase your skills, and you will increase both the number and the depth of your relationships.

As relationships build, emotions get stronger, and emotions open the subconscious trapdoor to decision-making. Since people make decisions based on emotions, the quality of your relationships will be a driving force and a key determinant in your success.

Remember that communication goes beyond the words you say. Your attitude, body language, communication style, and personal appearance are key elements in how successful you will be in your practice and are some of the core ideologies in building new relationships.

Relationship building will ultimately provide an unlimited stream of high-quality new patients for you to serve.

Get Creative

Soon, you'll have the tools to get to work on your yearly marketing calendar, and if you're going to design a yearly marketing calendar, you'll need to get creative so the energy around your promotions stays high. It's boring and unattractive to do the same old promotions over and over, so mix it up by choosing different aspects of practice and marketing to support with different events.

When you run an event-driven practice, you are constantly creating the next theme and agenda to go along with your events, and that imagination and innovation generates an energy field around yourself and your office. The expectation, excitement, and anticipation for the next event keep your patients on their toes and always trying to guess what you will do next.

How can you capture and demonstrate the fun you are having in your practice with your current patients? Will you have a blog or an events bulletin board to post articles, pictures, and testimonials from your past events to encourage all of your patients to participate? A monthly or quarterly newsletter can highlight recent events and promote future ones. Will you sponsor a short podcast, reporting on your events so your followers can learn and respond? Display the excitement, and encourage your current patients to share them with those they care about.

We're at our most creative when we realize that there are no limits to our imagination. Let your mind wander, and access your most powerful resources. Now consider, what makes your practice unique? How can those special qualities and characteristics of your practice be worked into your marketing and promotional events?

What makes your town special? Is there a way to customize the events so that they are congruent with your community? Open your thinking to any and all ideas. During team meetings, share ideas and brainstorm together so that everyone can contribute and take part in the creative process, and thereby feel like they have a stake in the success of the event.

Breaking bread together is universally enjoyed and appreciated, so serving refreshments at your events may be a nice added touch. The key is to create a happy and fun environment, and food and drink may be one of the little sparks that you need. You may want to be creative and choose refreshments that go along with the themes of your events.

For example, if you are holding a Healthy Food Party, you might serve organic cut vegetables with vegan dips, while for a Women's Night Of Indulgence, you may be better off with wine and chocolates. If you're doing an event for kids, you might serve yogurt bars, boxes of raisins, fruit and apple juice, while seniors might do better with little sandwiches or finger foods.

Experiment, break routines, and have fun. Envision your event before it actually takes place—what do you dream of, what does it look, sound, smell, taste, and feel like? How many people are there? If there were no rules and you could not fail, what would the event be like?

Now, let's explore how you could use The Event Driven Practice concept to fill your practice with great new patients. Remember, when you change and expand your beliefs toward abundance and do what needs to be done to serve more patients, you'll experience more miracles and create the practice and life of your dreams.

Plan a Yearly Marketing Calendar

Many successful practitioners plan their marketing calendars a year in advance. They do this to make marketing a priority and to allow time for this critical aspect of the practice. Planning your marketing events a year out requires organization and the right step-by-step instructions in order to make sure that all of your bases are covered.

By following this simple procedure, you will be able to plan your yearly marketing calendar before the year begins.

1) You'll need a large calendar that will serve as the office's marketing calendar for the year. Make sure there is enough room in each box to write event titles, action steps, reminders and other relevant information. If you like, you can design a large whiteboard for this purpose.

2) Aim for at least one or two events planned per month. Don't take on more than you can handle. Just because three events look great one month, doesn't mean you need to do them all. Figure out how many doctors and staff you need to make each event work so you can plan accurately. Don't bite off more than you can chew—plan each event carefully and give it your all. Besides—there's always next year!

3) Once you have chosen your events for the year, start deciding on the dates that each event will take place. For example, if you choose to host a New Year, New You Mastermind in your office, when will that take place? January 2nd? January 5th? January 23rd? What date works best with your office's schedule? How about with your community's calendar? Once you have chosen a date for each event, insert each of them into your marketing calendar.

4) After each event date has been written in your calendar, now it's time to plan each preparation milestone as well. For example, let's say you decide to host a New Year, New You Mastermind in your office on January 5th. About three and a half weeks prior to the workshop, customize and print enough flyers to be distributed to patients in your office, about 30 select inactive patients, as well as local gyms, community centers, and preschools in your community. This is also a good time to choose the 30 hand-picked inactive patients you feel would be great candidates for reactivation.

This means that somewhere around December 10th, you must write in your calendar "Customize and print New Year, New You flyers—enough for active patients, 30 inactive patients, and the community. Choose 30 inactive patients who are great candidates for reactivation."

About two and a half weeks before the date of the event, post the flyers at local gyms, community centers and preschools, and mail them out to the 30 hand-picked inactive patients whom you feel would be great candidates for reactivation. The more places you post your flyers, the more exposure you will gain. Post the flyer in your practice, and hand it out to patients as they leave the office. Around December 17th, plot in your calendar "Post New Year, New You flyers in the office, local gyms, community centers and preschools. Mail them to the 30 inactive patients." Get the idea? As responses come in, decide if you need to invite more people or engage more local entities to fill your program to your satisfaction.

Then, continue plotting the rest of your preparation dates. Ten days before the event, call each of the 30 inactive patients who were sent flyers to invite them to attend this interactive workshop, and purchase envelopes, stamps, and paper (if you don't have it on hand). Around December 26th, write these preparation steps into your calendar.

Continue plotting your preparation steps until you are finished with the event. Repeat this process for each event you choose to host throughout the year. If these directions are followed, you will have a smooth and efficient preparation and planning process.

By January 3, confirm all participants. Have a CA call and confirm each guest using the following script:

"Hi, this is Leslie from Dr. Perman's office. I'm calling to confirm your attendance at our New Year, New You Mastermind."

Then restate the date and time, and give the office address and clear directions. Briefly reiterate the intent of the workshop: "Remember, Mr.

Patient, this is a fun and interactive workshop, where our goal is to provide you with a better insight into getting the most out of yourself in the new year, and teach you some natural and effective ways to stay well and prevent symptoms and illnesses."

Ask if they have any questions, to reduce any miscommunications and allow the event to flow smoothly. Double check to make sure they have your phone number.

On January 4, purchase all refreshments to be served during the event. And finally, on January 5, set up the office—it's show time!

Remember that you'll need to follow up with all guests, get feedback, and make sure they had a great experience. It's all part of relationship building!

Make your calendar work for YOUR practice. If there is a month that offers four events, but your practice can only handle two, it will create overwhelm. Doing too many events can have the opposite effect and be detrimental to your practice. Be realistic, and develop a healthy balance that generates sufficient new patient flow but doesn't stress your office or your team.

Finding Balance

Aim for two to three internal events each month on a consistent basis. They should be enjoyable and profitable. As you know, it is essential to attract new patients and to dramatically increase your patient retention. Therefore, events should be targeted to your active and inactive patient base as well as their friends and families.

If you are a sole practitioner, it is essential to space out your events so that your practice can run efficiently. However, if you have multiple doctors in the office, it may be easier to do more events. It's important to be aware of your capacity so that you can find the right balance between the number of events you plan each month and your daily schedule. While every doctor wants a busy practice, set reasonable standards.

Staying Organized

Organization is a vital key to success—especially in an event-driven practice. Staying organized will allow you to maximize the impact each event has on your practice and keep you on the path toward growth.

Assign each event its own folder to be filed away in your Event Driven Practice filing cabinet. All notes, documents, receipts, and outlines should be filed away in their respective folders.

Debrief after each event to make distinctions about what worked, what didn't, and what can be done differently to ensure the success of the event in the future.

This keeps the communication flowing among the staff and helps you plan ahead. When you are ready to do that specific event again, you will be able to read your notes and tweak your plans so you focus on the factors that will make your event as successful as possible.

Plotting your dates correctly, finding the right balance with the number of events you choose to do, and staying organized will ensure your success as streams of new patients begin flowing toward you.

Now that you understand the basic format for planning and creating effective promotions, let's talk about two broad categories of promotions—internal promotions and external promotions.

Internal Promotions

Internal promotions are centered on your office and your current patients. They are usually publicized through your office as a home base, and many of the participants are current patients and their guests. The New Year New You Mastermind is an example of an internal promotion.

There are many advantages to running promotions on the premises of your office. First, there is no additional rental charge, and you have complete control of the facility. There is no stress or pressure on the timing of setting up, so you can work at your own pace and still be confident you'll get everything done. Also, it's good to have events at your office so people who are attracted to you find you, and see how nice and convenient your location is for them.

There aren't many drawbacks—sometimes there are parking issues, and once in a while some food or drink gets spilled on the rug, but mostly, your office is a controlled environment that can be adapted to run successful events.

There are dozens of internal promotions you can do, from playing the three-a-day game to applying family health histories, from creating a testimonials book or wall to sponsoring patient appreciation dinners, from holiday celebrations to charity drives. They engage the community, position you as an advanced citizen, and make you the go-to chiropractor for people who become familiar with your name and your office.

Patient Appreciation Days and Dinners

Let's talk a little about Patient Appreciation Days and Patient Appreciation Dinners.

The more you show your appreciation for patients, the more opportunity you get to serve them. Dr. Hoffman says, "Reward the behavior you want," so if patients feel rewarded, it helps you to shape their behavior by increasing emotional charge.

When people feel good around you and are treated well by you, it's not unreasonable to expect that they will tend to return the compliment.

A great way to do this is with a Patient Appreciation Day, where you schedule a day where you offer complimentary services to current and new patients, either just as a gift or in exchange for a small donation to a worthy cause. Be careful to know the law in your area, as some jurisdictions may not permit complimentary services without appropriate disclaimers, and sometimes not at all. In this situation, have patients pay you a small donation you can contribute to a charity, and that will be legal most places.

Many doctors use Patient Appreciation Days to set records in daily office visit volume, to gain experience seeing many more people than usual in a single day. They also generate referrals, and most doctors who run these promotions report that they most often attract high-quality new patients.

A popular derivative of Patient Appreciation Day is a Patient Appreciation Dinner, where you sponsor a dinner party where you or a guest speaker presents to a handpicked group of your patients and their guests. Breaking bread together and then making a good case for engaging chiropractic care is a powerful combination. Usually you would pick a restaurant owned by a patient so the networking is increased, but if that's not available, pick one of the better places in town, always with a private room to have your meeting within your party where the speaker educates the crowd, hopefully to inspire the guests to opt in on your care.

After the speaker closes, the doctors and team should fan out to engage the group, making sure they were entertained and offering them the opportunity to begin care. Part of the team preparation should include some role-playing in this scenario so it's comfortable and familiar at the dinner.

Be careful not to allow these events to degenerate into pure marketing—they are designed to be fueled by the positivity and love demonstrated by you for your patients, without whom your practice and life would be very different. Expressing gratitude is a high form of communication, and showing your patients how you feel cements your relationship with them.

External Promotions

There are also many kinds of events you can plan outside your office. They take similar attention to detail, but require engaging the community more and targeting individuals, businesses, other professionals, and groups that you can serve, and can help you get your message out.

There are many advantages to doing external promotions. They open up fresh referral pools, spread your legend beyond your physical boundaries, help you experience new and interesting people and adventures, and most of all, give you the opportunity to serve an ever-expanding number of people.

External promotions often take more work and planning than internal promotions, but they offer more public exposure and more variety to keep your new patient process fresh and effective.

When you establish a foundation of internal promotions and a variety of external promotions to fill in your yearly marketing calendar, you create certainty without risking boredom.

There are myriad types of external promotions, including community events, advertising and direct mail, social media marketing, surveys, telemarketing, charity drives, writing health columns and articles, becoming a company chiropractor, and many, many others.

Spinal Screenings

Other than lecturing, which we talked about in Chapter 4, perhaps one of the fastest ways to create a flow of new patients into your practice is to conduct spinal screenings. It is a time- and cost-efficient means of generating large numbers of new patients.

The purpose of a Spinal Screening is to introduce the public to chiropractic care. You are there to establish the role that chiropractic can play in meeting their health care needs, now and in the future ... and, the acquisition of the new patients that come as a result are a bonus!

If you are truly going out to spread the word of chiropractic, the higher purpose we so often speak about, you will be rewarded by the great feeling you get, and you'll attract some new patients, too.

A Spinal Screening is not successful or unsuccessful based upon the number of examinations you conduct. It is successful if you accomplish what you set out to do ... tell the world about chiropractic. From our vantage point, we notice that doctors who conduct a Spinal Screening are often elated or depressed by the number of people who "sign-up" to come in.

That suggests that the intent was solely to get more new patients, to hype the practice and make more money. This may seem legitimate, but lacks in the higher purpose of someone who is sincerely focused on the benefit that chiropractic care can have on humanity.

Many doctors realize that in the course of the following weeks after the event, the number of new patients processed by the office was dramatically increased, but the new patients did not necessarily come directly from the screening.

The point is, what goes around, comes around—what you put out, you get back. So, remember to conduct the spinal screening with focus, energy, care, love for chiropractic, and a higher purpose. Then, if you can, release the outcome, trust that the right results will manifest, and see what happens.

Anytime you present yourself in public, you, by the very nature of who you are, have an opportunity to turn on the new patient faucet. One of the most fun and exciting parts of a screening is that you never know what will happen with these new people you will meet. Many patients I connected with at such gatherings became regular patients and made numerous referrals, often a dozen or more over the years.

There are numerous forms a screening can take, with shades of difference in presentation and strategy—there are scoliosis screenings, stress screenings, posture screenings, health fairs, expos, mall shows, trade shows, mall kiosks—there are many configurations that you can adapt the following procedures to fit.

Where To Conduct Your Screenings

Here are a few places to consider when you plan your spinal screening:

1. Health fairs

2. Health clubs

3. Health food stores

4. Shopping malls

5. Business and industry

6. Flea markets

7. County fairs

8. Street fairs

Spinal screenings conducted at health fairs, health clubs, and health food stores tend to yield the best results. They attract people who already possess a health "consciousness" to begin with. You may have a greater influence on people who are already interested in not only getting well ... but staying well!

Getting Started

1. Contact your local Chamber of Commerce, service organizations, health clubs, and local charities and find out where and when future events are scheduled.

2. Personally visit local health clubs, gyms, and spas to determine if they are willing to sponsor a free spinal screening for their clientele. Do your best to speak directly with the owner or decision-maker, and remember to emphasize the benefits they'll get from this event.

3. Aim for one screening each quarter, and register early to secure the best booth location. Some offices can handle a more rigorous schedule—experiment to see what works best in your office.

4. Register for all major annual events as soon as possible.

5. Have a booth you can be proud of and that represents chiropractic in the best possible light. Appearance is critical, so be sure the booth is attractive and eye-catching. Don't skimp!

6. While it is best to have a NeuroInfiniti, Insight, or Posture Analyzer, you can conduct a screening without them. You do want to educate the

people you meet, so you may want to bring along an adjusting table, a plastic spine, some charts of the brain, spine, and nerve system, appropriate literature and pamphlets, and perhaps even some videos that provide short and simple explanations about chiropractic care.

7. Bring some chairs for potential patients to sit on as you explain the benefits of chiropractic. Also, bring your appointment book, appointment cards, professional cards, screening information forms, and pens.

8. A properly attired professional chiropractic assistant is a huge asset.

Sample Dialogues

What to say and how to "close" are obviously of great importance to the success of the screening. Here are some ideas for you to personalize and develop:

"Mrs. Jones, the brief examination we just conducted reveals that most of your spine and nerve system seem to be functioning reasonably well— however, the exam did point out a few potential problem areas.

"When I tested your movement, I found your lower back out of alignment (or whatever you found), and there is evidence of nerve interference that calls for some further testing. This could be causing the problem you reported."

Or, if the patient is not experiencing any symptoms, direct your discussion toward brain stress, ranges of motion, tenderness upon palpation, objective findings from the technology on hand, or an introduction to wellness.

"In my opinion, it would be worth your consideration to have a complete examination of your spine and nerve system to determine your level of brain stress and how you may benefit from chiropractic care. This is strictly your option. It is impossible for me to really determine the extent of a potential problem without a full examination, taking the time and using the right equipment, but from what I see so far, you would learn a lot you need to know about your body from this exam.

"Normally, a complete chiropractic exam costs between $75 and $150. (We suggest you select a fee that you feel comfortable with, but give up the need to give your services away. If your usual policy is to offer a complimentary consultation, it's fine to offer that.)

"If, for any reason, the exam indicates the need for further testing, that will be discussed with you in advance, and you will have the option to proceed or re-evaluate at that time. Rest assured that no one will ever talk you into anything you don't want to do.

"Mrs. Jones, it is also important to me that you not make an appointment simply because it is difficult to say no. Please, accept this opportunity only if you are genuinely interested in discovering the degree of interference in your nerve system and your level of brain stress ... is that fair? When would it be convenient for you to come in for the examination? Do you prefer mornings or afternoons?"

Follow-Up Procedure

The follow-up procedure is designed for people who were receptive at the screening, but who were not ready to make an appointment at that time. You can call them a few days after the screening and, in a gentle and respectful way, tell them that it was a pleasure to meet them, and ask them if it would be okay to send them a periodic mailing that would be of interest. Stay in contact with them, because some people need more time or more exposures to you in order to feel comfortable enough to get started.

In summary, screenings are a very effective way to demonstrate chiropractic to a large number of people and, as a result, to fill your office with lots of new patients.

Hiring the Right Public Relations Director

Running an event-driven practice isn't the easiest task—especially if you are working alone. That's why it is always best to have someone orchestrating these events with you and your practice. You might already have the perfect person working for you, or, you might need to hire someone on a part-time or per-project basis in order to help you implement the events that are attractive to you.

Either way, it is important to remember that personality, organization, persistence, and enthusiasm are required to properly execute an event-driven practice.

If you already have someone working for you that might be perfect for this new position, ask yourself the following questions:

1. If this person takes on this new task, will I need to hire someone else to cover his or her old tasks in the office?

2. Does this person have both an outgoing personality and the ability to stay focused and organized?

3. Before I change this person's position and tasks, am I committed to the concept of the Event Driven Practice, and am I prepared to support this person in any way needed?

These are important questions to ask yourself in order to ensure that your office runs as efficiently as possible. If you have to hire someone else to cover the everyday office tasks, make sure you go through the hiring process while your new PR director has time to train the new addition to your team. This way, your office continues to run smoothly.

The most important part of this process is your desire and willingness to run regular promotions. So many doctors like the idea of running an event-driven practice, so they hire someone to handle it all for them and then step away, but that rarely works. Regular promotion requires the attention and energy of the doctor. In fact, it is suggested that the doctor and PR director meet regularly to touch base and discuss all of the happenings within the practice. This way, the doctor can hold the PR director accountable and make sure that events are being planned in the right way—with the detailed planning of an event-driven practice, it is vital that the doctor be involved and be kept in the loop with everything.

If you are thinking about hiring someone else for this specialized job in your office, ask yourself the following questions to help you on your hiring journey:

1. Do I have a patient who has a great personality and is dedicated to me and to chiropractic?

2. Do I have a friend or family member who would be perfect for this part-time position?

3. Do I have any people in my personal and professional database I could e-mail or call for a referral?

Often, the right person to hire is right under your nose—you just don't know it yet. For the next two weeks, concentrate on each patient who comes into your office. Ask yourself if they would be a great candidate to be the PR director of your office. If the answer is yes, then whether or not they have a job, simply ask them, "By the way, would you be curious about a part-time job being my public relations director?" See what their answer is—you never know! You just might find the perfect person this way.

Friends and family can also become trusted and capable staff members. They typically have a vested interest in the success of your practice due to your relationship.

Ask the people in your personal and professional database, throughout your sphere of influence, for recommendations.

If you need to, place an ad in your local paper or job posting website. You'll have to screen more carefully, but you can still find great candidates that way.

Ultimately, the right person for the job is the one who will help you fill your marketing calendar with productive events so your practice is fun and educational and prosperous.

You may want to hire someone on a ninety-day trial basis, to ensure that they are the right person for the job. Event planning takes skill and personality that not everyone has—so, allow for a reasonable learning curve, but trust your intuition and work toward having the best possible player in that position.

The Power of Media

Once you have your PR Director hired and trained, you'll want to use the power of the media to help you broaden the radius of your appeal. In fact, the more you do, the more exposure you will gain and the better results you will have.

Local television, radio, newspapers, websites, and blogs are always seeking new and exciting community events they can list and recommend. With health and wellness now being one of the hottest topics of conversation, if you are serving your community by providing education on the most popular health and wellness topics out there, you can often get coverage from the media. By reaching out to the various media outlets, you can tell them who you are and what you have to offer, and some will be curious about you and take the next steps.

The Internet is the best way to search for local media outlets. Google your city or town's name, along with the word "television station" then "radio station" then "newspaper," etc. You might even know most of the popular sources because you probably watch, read, and listen to your local media as your source for information as well.

Once you have gathered a list of media outlets to contact by doing a little research online, you then have to discover and connect with a contact person at each of these places. You might already know someone in this industry—a patient, friend, or family member. Engage them—let them know what you can offer them and how it will benefit the community. Keep it brief, focused, and relevant, and if there isn't any interest, accept that and maintain the relationship—you may appeal better to them next time, so ensure there is a next time with courtesy and respect.

Submit a press release to your contact person at each media outlet. Press releases get published when they are perceived to be relevant, in other words, that people can relate to the content and be interested or entertained by it.

For example, let's say that National Osteoporosis Prevention Month is considered to be a current event in the month of October. Therefore, during that month, provide an Osteoporosis Prevention workshop in your office, and inform the media about this complimentary service you are providing to the community.

Press releases typically state who, what, where, when, and why. In a few minutes we're going to look at some sample letters, press releases, and flyers, which you can customize and e-mail, fax, mail, or post on social media, and follow up with the people on your list individually. Keep expanding your list, and keep sending press releases to your list about the various events you will be hosting in your office and how they relate to current events that will help the community. Being thorough and persistent is key!

Here is a sample follow-up dialogue that a member of your staff (or you) can use when following up with the contact person at each media outlet.

"Hi, can I please speak to Mr. Young? Hello, Mr. Young, my name is Susie, and I'm calling on behalf of Dr. John Brown of the Brown Health and Wellness Center. I'm calling to follow up on a press release that I sent you via e-mail on December 4 regarding the Osteoporosis Lecture Dr. Brown will be presenting at his office next week. Do you remember if you received the press release I am referring to?"

If the contact person says no, simply ask if you can send it again and give a follow-up time that they can expect to hear back from you. If yes, continue.

"This event is special because we are dedicated to educating the community on health issues like osteoporosis, to help them understand what they can do to be as healthy as possible.

"It's going to be a great event. It's open to the community at no cost, and I was calling to see if you could help us spread the word." (Wait for confirmation.) "Oh, that would be great. If you have any questions in the meantime, my name is Susie, and I would be happy to answer any questions you may have. You can reach me at 555-5555. Have a nice day! Good-bye."

Media outlets receive hundreds of these, so you have to follow up to improve your chances of being noticed, until you establish a reputation. Remember to make sure that you focus on the fact that you are helping the community.

If your contact person sounds intrigued and interested, keep your conversation moving and try to develop a relationship with the person. Over time, this contact could potentially help you spread the word for all of your events—which would be a great way to consistently gain exposure.

Since communication is always one of the keys to success, make sure you communicate like an expert, not a salesperson. In fact, you aren't selling anything—you are simply informing the media about providing a public service of sharing your expertise on important subjects. Educate your community and gain as much exposure as you can. The rewards will come.

Sample Materials

Now, let's look at some examples of letters, press releases, and materials you can use to operate your promotions. You can mix and match, based on what appeals to you, or write your own, using some of these ideas to prime your creative pump.

Sample Marketing Calendar

JANUARY	FEBRUARY	MARCH	APRIL	MAY	JUNE
PEAK PERFORMANCE THE SIX FACETS OF HEALTH WOMEN'S WELLNESS WORKSHOP HAT/COAT DRIVE	HEALTHY HEART MONTH YOU ARE WHAT YOU EAT! VALENTINE'S DAY DINNER RAFFLE	NIGHT OF INDULGENCE SPRING CLEAN AND EAT CHOCOLATE!! ALLERGY RELIEF NATURALLY!!	INTERNATIONAL JOKE DAY SPRING DETOX BACK SAFETY AND INJURY PREVENTION WEEK	STAY FIT WHILE YOU SIT YOGA IN THE PARK WELL MAMA DAY	STRESS SURVEYS STRESS MANAGEMENT WEEK WELL DADDY DAY
JULY	AUGUST	SEPTEMBER	OCTOBER	NOVEMBER	DECEMBER
FREEDOM OF HEALTH CHOICE SUMMER BAKING CONTEST HAWAIIAN LUAU	HYDRATION AWARENESS MONTH KID'S HEALTH AND SAFETY DAY SCHOOL SUPPLIES DRIVE	FIVE-A-DAY WEEK WALK FOR HEALTH FINDING THE FOUNTAIN OF YOUTH LECTURE SERIES	HEALTHY HALLOWEEN VEGETARIAN COOK-OFF MONSTER'S BALL/PATIENT APPRECIATION DINNER	THANKSGIVING FOOD DRIVE MOVIE NIGHT VETERANS WEEK	TOY AND BOOK DRIVE PATIENT RECOGNITION WEEK FORTUNE COOKIE DAY

This is an example of a yearly marketing calendar. You can see that I picked three events for each month—adjust the content and number of promotions to your capacity and practice philosophy. Here are some ideas for fliers, ads, and press releases.

Women's Wellness Workshop

This invitation announces a women's wellness workshop.

Women's Wellness Workshop

Dr. _____ from *<name of practice>* will be presenting a Women's Wellness Workshop (For Women Only) on *<date>* at *<location of practice>* from *<time>*

The purpose of this workshop is to share natural and effective methods of dealing with women's health issues. Topics include heart healthy habits, avoiding (or dealing with) osteoporosis, anti-aging techniques, and much more.

This workshop is complimentary for women in the community, however, seating is limited. Please call <*name of CA*> at: (___) ___-____ for more information.

Contact Person:
Company Name:
Telephone Number:
Fax Number:
E-mail Address:
Website address:

Sample Press Release—Osteoporosis Workshop

This is an example of a press release announcing your osteoporosis workshop, timed to match up with National Osteoporosis Prevention month.

SAMPLE PRESS RELEASE—OSTEOPOROSIS WORKSHOP

FOR IMMEDIATE RELEASE

(NAME OF PRACTICE) HELPS THE COMMUNITY PREVENT OSTEOPOROSIS IN AN EDUCATIONAL WORKSHOP CALLED:

STICKS AND STONES MAY BREAK MY BONES BUT OSTEOPOROSIS WILL NEVER HARM ME!

(Date of workshop)
(Time frame of workshop)
(Location and address)

October is National Osteoporosis Prevention Month

(Insert your home town and state)—(Insert today's date, year)—The National Osteoporosis Foundation says over 44 million Americans suffer from osteoporosis, considered a major public threat to more than half of those 55 years or older. (http://www.nof.org/osteoporosis/diseasefacts.htm)

(Name of practice) is hosting an osteoporosis awareness workshop presented by (Dr. First Name Last name) called "Sticks and Stones May Break My Bones but Osteoporosis will Never Harm Me!" This talk will explain how to address this serious problem through simple, lifestyle-related changes.

(Dr. Last Name), a local wellness doctor, said, "I'm committed to educating our community on health issues like osteoporosis. Our free workshops are designed to help people learn how to get well and stay well naturally."

Local Contact
Dr. (your name here)
Practice name here
Your address
Your Phone #
Your E-mail address

National Injury Prevention Month

And this is a letter to set up a talk about National Injury Prevention month.

Dear HR or Safety Coordinator,

In honor of National Injury Prevention Month, we invite you to take advantage of an opportunity to have Dr. _____ speak to your employees on Back Safety and Injury Prevention.

As part of our community awareness program, we are offering this opportunity to select businesses in the area at no cost. The workshop is about 45 minutes in length, and Dr. _____ will teach your team how to properly lift, bend, push, and pull to reduce injury on the job and at home. This then reduces the impact on your company due to lost time and productivity.

Dr. _____ speaks regularly to local businesses on health, wellness, and safety topics. His mission is to educate and empower as many people as possible to experience their optimal health potential.

To set up a time for Dr. _____ to come in and provide a workshop for your employees, please call *<name of CA handling calls>* at (___) ___-____.

Yours in good health,

Flier for Physical Fitness Fair

Here's copy for a flier on sponsoring a Fitness Fair:

(Name of Practice)'s
Physical Fitness Fair
(Sample Schedule)
Saturday, May 2nd from noon to 3 PM

- **12:00—12:15 PM**—Welcome to all guests, schedule, price sheet, and raffle tickets handed out.

- **12:15—12:45 PM**—Basic Yoga class with (name of yoga instructor).

- **12:50—1:20 PM**—Weight Training Workshop—The Dos and "Don'ts of Successful Weight Training with (name of personal trainer).

- **1:30—2:00 PM**—Beginner Pilates with (name of Pilates instructor).

- **2:00—2:40 PM**—Each instructor is available for one-on-one consultations and demonstrations. Exercise equipment is for sale for a reduced fee (see price sheet for details).

- **2:40—3:00 PM**—Winning raffle ticket is picked by (name of doctor) and the winner is announced. The winner must be present to receive the gift basket. If he or she is not present, there will be another raffle ticket drawn until a winner is determined.

Letter for National Stress Awareness Month

This is a letter promoting you to present at an accounting firm on stress reduction.

Name of Accounting Firm
Address
City, State, Zip Code
Date

Dear (Human Resource/General Manager),

In honor of National Stress Awareness Month and the end of tax season, we invite you to take advantage of an opportunity to have Dr. _____ speak to your staff on the topic of Stress Management. As part of our community awareness program, this service is provided free of charge.

The workshop is about 45 minutes in length, and Dr. _____ will speak about ways to identify physical, emotional, and chemical stress, and help people gain a better understanding of how stress affects their overall health. Dr. _____ will also discuss how stress can be minimized in the workplace and at home.

As an added bonus to the CPAs, Accountants, executive, and support staff, we would be happy to bring a massage therapist with us to perform chair massages while the staff listens to the workshop. Now that's what we call stress management!

Dr. _____ speaks regularly to local businesses on health, wellness, and safety topics. His mission is to educate and empower as many people as possible to experience their optimal health potential.

To schedule a time for Dr. _____ to come in for a workshop, please call (name of CA handling calls) at (OFFICE PHONE HERE).

Yours in good health,
(Name of Practice)

PS. These valuable workshops are presented free of charge as a public service. Please call to schedule a time to discuss how Dr. (doctor's name) can help your team decrease stress and improve productivity.

Letter for Pediatric Lecture

This is a letter you can use to set up lectures for staff and parents at schools or day care centers.

Name of Doctor
Address
City, State, Zip Code
Date

Dear (Name of Preschool/Daycare Director),

In honor of Healthy Child Day, please accept our gift of having Dr. _____ speak to your staff and parents on the popular topic of Raising Healthy Children in a Not-So-Healthy World. As part of our community awareness program, this service is provided at no charge.

The workshop is about 45 minutes in length, and Dr. _____ will speak about the many health and wellness issues that parents face today for their children—such as ear infections, colic, bedwetting, antibiotic use and abuse, ADD/ADHD, developing wellness habits and much, much more.

Since you are a daycare center/preschool, on occasion you probably invite the parents of the children that attend your school to a parents' evening, where guest speakers present workshops about the hottest topics affecting children. We take responsibility for being community thought leaders on pediatric health and well-being. Please let us share this all-natural approach with you and the families you serve.

Dr. _____ speaks regularly to organizations on health, wellness, and safety topics. (His/Her) mission is to educate and empower as many people as possible to experience their optimal health potential.

To set up a time for Dr. _____ to come in and provide a workshop to your staff during a staff meeting or parents during a parents' evening, please call (name of CA handling calls) at (xxx) xxx-xxxx.

Yours for better health,

Random Acts of Kindness

You can be as creative as you like—this is copy for a flier on promoting Random Acts of Kindness and inviting people to purchase a gift certificate for health and wellness services.

Random Acts of Kindness ...

Give out compliments . . . Smile

Accept . . . Let someone go ahead of you in line

Have patience . . . Send notes of gratitude and appreciation

Send love notes . . . Hold a door open for someone

Start a conversation with a stranger . . . Visit a nursing home

Send an anonymous gift

The Gift of Health for the Holiday Season ...

(Name of Practice)

To: _____

From: _____

This Gift Certificate Entitles You to a

Holiday Wellness Package!
Your Wellness Package Includes:

A diet and nutritional review

Suggestions for relevant and appropriate exercises

A stress evaluation including a chiropractic exam and a positive thinking
survey that provides guidance for healthier thoughts and emotions

A one-hour massage

Authorized Signature: _____

Expiration Date: _____

Name: _____

Phone Number:_____

Lose-a-Rama

This is copy for a flier about a Lose-a-Rama weight reduction contest. These are great new patient attractors, and the clientele you attract are often ripe to make big change, and that makes them receptive to your leadership.

1st Annual Lose-a-Rama Weight Reduction Contest!

Name of your office here

Contest: (DATE RANGE)

Kickoff Party: (DATE and TIME)

Phone: (000) 000-0000

123 Any Street, City, State

Rules and Regulations

All contestants must be present for the kickoff party held on (date of kickoff party) in addition to the grand finale celebration held on (date of grand finale celebration).

All contestants must weigh in once a week, at their convenience, to record weekly weight, scheduled prior to beginning the contest. Contestants must agree to lose weight in a healthy manner, through proper diet and exercise.

Local Contact Dr. (your name here) Practice name here Your address Your Phone # Your E-mail address

There are so many options, it will help you to organize or chunk your marketing so you know where your attention is best invested. We'll be talking about the mechanisms of the new patient machine in Chapter 8, but for now, let's look at a tool that can keep you focused on promoting yourself consistently and effectively.

Five-by-Five Marketing

Let's talk about a fun and productive marketing process called Five-by-Five Marketing.

As many of you know, as a coach I believe in surrounding myself with and learning from experts, and to help me with my writing, marketing, and publicity, I work with Bill and Steve Harrison's Quantum Leap. It's fun being on the receiving side of seminars and coaching for a change, and a recent program featured Jack Canfield, one of the most popular and successful authors of our time.

Mr. Canfield was extremely open and generous in discussing his ascent to the top of the writing field from his origins as a schoolteacher, and taught us a hundred useful things, some of which I may have already known but had reconfirmed, others I got to experience for the first time—not the least of which is… we need to be willing to persist and work hard enough to earn the successes we desire.

In talking about how he and Mark Victor Hansen launched the Chicken Soup series, which has sold over 500 million copies worldwide, he revealed a tool they used daily to keep themselves pushing forward, which he simply referred to as "Five By Five." It is elegant in its simplicity and relevant to any kind of marketing and promotion, so I thought I would adapt it to the chiropractic practice so you can flood your office with all the new patients you prefer.

Just create a five-by-five grid, and down the left-hand side, write examples of your target market, in chiropractic language, your ideal, favorite types of patients. Then, complete the chart by writing in the adjacent boxes five strategies you could use to engage, attract, or convert these types of patients. For example:

Young mothers	Talk at PTA	Tupperware party	Article on raising a healthy family	Network with mothers in the practice	Post remarks on popular mothers' blog
Kids	Talk at school	Scoliosis screening	Kids' Health Newsletter	Visit martial arts dojo	E-mail kids' health tip of the week
Golfers	Talk at golf club	Golfer's night	List of Healthy Golfing Tips	Recruit golf pro from local club	Ask for referral from fellow golfer
Low back patients	Healthy Lifting Class	Low Back support group	Newsletter on avoiding low back injury	Take a local doctor to lunch	Send letter about new low back approach
Seniors	Anti-Aging Lecture	Seniors Mixer	Article on Healthy Habits for Seniors	Visit local seniors homes	Send gift card for referral

Once you have your five-by-five menu assembled, commit to a certain number of efforts every day—whether you do one, three, five, or more marketing approaches each day, your practice will grow, usually in proportion to the amount of energy you invest.

The trick to this strategy is in the consistency—yes, you may take some action at times, but are you dedicated to a schedule of performance that holds you to a higher standard of execution? Like the three-a-day game we talked about in Chapter 2, the power of these methods is in doing it every day. As you gather momentum, sand the rough edges off your skills and become a master.

For example, let's say you consider young families ideal patients. What are some action steps you could take to attract them? You could ask other families in your office for referrals, plan a talk for young families in your office, schedule a "Tupperware party" where a patient invites several young families to their house for a gathering you sponsor, engage other professionals who serve young families, or create a strategic alliance with merchants in your town who cater to young families.

If you picked five types of ideal patients, and developed five ways to market to each of them, you would have a variety of different fun things you could do; some more involved, and others requiring nothing more than a brief conversation to attract the people you most like to take care of.

In Chapter 8, we're going to complete our discussion of How To Target Your Ideal Patient, and when you get crystal clarity about the types of patients you want to attract, then this five-by-five marketing approach is perfect for turning those intentions into reality. List your five favorite kinds of new patients, develop five marketing approaches for each, and then just pick the number of tactics you plan on applying each day, week, or month.

I'm grateful to Jack Canfield for sharing this powerful technique. You never know where the great ideas will come from. Keep your mind open and your intentions clear, accept every opportunity to enrich your internal map, and take action on what you learn. That's how we grow, inside the skin and in our practices.

We'll also be going into greater depth with the concept of the marketing calendar in Chapter 8, so as you compile new patient attraction techniques that resonate with you, start thinking about where you will insert them into your schedule and how they fit into the grand scheme of your marketing for the year. Gaining this kind of perspective helps you use the natural momentum of your growth to keep your practice moving forward, serving more people and making a bigger difference on your community.

For now, get your feet wet with one or more of these promotional ideas— whether you plan an internal event like a Patient Appreciation Day, or an external event like a health fair or screening, there are potential new patients everywhere you look, if you only develop the skills to engage them so you can serve them.

Points to Remember

1. Develop an event-driven practice—it's entertaining, productive, and the variety will constantly refresh your marketing and keep it interesting and fun for you and your team.

2. Your practice rises and falls on your ability to create relationships— relate, reassure, reinforce, and react.

Actions to Take

1. Start to compile a marketing calendar with numerous different types of promotions so you gain experience in different methods of promoting yourself and your practice.

2. Delegate aspects of your marketing to talented and competent teammates to increase the energy without overloading your own schedule.

Questions to Ponder

1. If you have already established a consistent event-driven approach, what has the impact been? Why would you recommend or not recommend this practice style to other chiropractors?

2. Where could you expand or refine your marketing to include more fruitful events, and eliminate less productive ones?

Chapter 5 offered you broad exposure to the different types of promotions you can run, inside and outside your office. In Chapter 6, we'll be tackling Internet marketing and social media, so fasten your seat belt.

CHAPTER 6
Internet Marketing

This chapter is designed to introduce you to the amazing opportunities available with the Internet, through online marketing, content distribution, networking, and relationship building.

I've spent thousands of hours surfing the net, and I've only scratched the tiniest nick into the surface of the cyberuniverse. It would be overly optimistic to think that within the confines of this chapter I could present the entirety of your necessary insight into this remarkable asset.

Rather, I will add dimension to your understanding by singling out some relatively easy methods to improve your results and attract new patients every day through the Internet, and we'll mention many different tools you can use to expand your influence and increase the number of people you touch and serve.

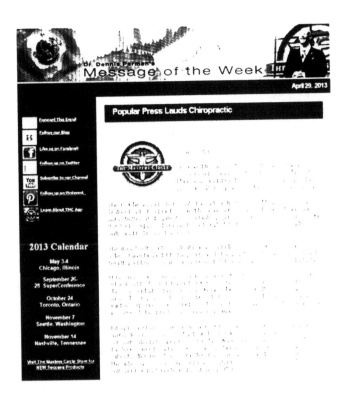

For example, many of you receive my free Message of the Week, published Monday mornings since September 8, 1997, at the time of this writing over 900 consecutive weeks. If you are not currently receiving it and wish to, please let me know.

At the very beginning I was green and inexperienced, even by that day's standards. I felt I had something to say, a decade into my chiropractic coaching career, and I needed a way to express myself and expand my service to our profession.

All I knew about the Internet was America Online, so I searched for all the chiropractors who were signed up on AOL, about 1,200 at the time, and used them to start prospecting to build my mailing list, my first opportunity to ask people to opt in. Many were not interested, some unsubscribed, but many others became clients, members, customers, and friends over the years, even a few who have been with me since the very beginning.

It's tough to guess how many impressions have been made by this column—my mailing list, referred to as a "platform" in contemporary marketing jargon, has been between one and five thousand over the years, and besides those I e-mail directly to those subscribers, many doctors read them at staff meetings, hand them out to patients, ask for permission to reprint them or forward them, and post them on social media. I've received feedback from twelve countries. If you figure even 1,000 impressions from each edition, it's about a million times people got to read my words, and it could be five or ten times that or more, a humbling thought.

That's why I keep my standards high when writing for my cherished readers like you. It's like the old story about Joe DiMaggio, the all-time great Hall Of Fame center fielder for the New York Yankees in the years surrounding World War II.

An enthusiastic young reporter was interviewing DiMag, and asked him, "Joltin' Joe, why do you play so hard?" The Yankee Clipper replied without missing a beat, "It's because I can't take the chance that someone is seeing me play for the first or the last time."

I feel the same way. I only want to put out the highest quality coaching and products, those I can be proud of and confident that my customers will be pleased with, in case it's the first or last time I get to serve them, to make or leave the best possible impression. I want the very best for them, for you, at all times. Learning to use the Internet as a source of new patients requires the same meticulous scruples, because once you put something out into cyberspace, it's unlikely you'll be able to take it back.

Ask any of the politicians who edged over that line and discovered that it was a cliff they were stepping off, plummeting to an untimely demise.

For that reason, you'll want to carefully consider any communication you put out; make sure it really says what you want it to say, and also to protect yourself legally and ethically, and avoid any misunderstanding that could be inconvenient or embarrassing, or even unwittingly hurtful. My dad, the late Dr. William Perman, may he rest in peace, taught me that it's usually better to be sorry you didn't than sorry you did—in other words, discretion is the better part of valor.

Learning to use the power of the information superhighway is one of the most useful and productive assets you have available, but the risk of wasted time, energy, and capital looms large. Choose an amount of time, based on your current level of mastery, that you are willing to commit to online research and marketing. It may take some of us a short while to figure out the rhythm, but soon enough you'll feel comfortable with the technology and will be ready to delve into this fascinating field of promotion.

Before you attempt to embark on this amazing journey, some preparation time is in order—online communication has its own language, its own timing, its own etiquette and rules structure.

For example, something as simple as accidentally leaving the caps lock key on your keyboard makes any experienced online communicator THINK YOU ARE SHOUTING—or, that you are too lame to realize you have the caps lock key on. Only write in capital letters for very strong emphasis, and please use that privilege sparingly.

Much of the research I did to prepare this chapter came from years of daily experience, simply searching the net, as most of you have also done many times. What you may not realize is that there's an evolving science to positioning yourself so someone looking for what you do finds you.

Using The Internet—Receiving and Sending

Using the Internet has two giant categories of utilization—receiving and sending. Receiving includes research, information gathering, reading and studying, tapping into databases and surveys to interpret trends, and any way you can use the vast resources to collect relevant data, from a telephone number to an entire encyclopedia to a hundred articles on some infinitesimal detail of anatomy or physiology that gives you the cherry on top of your health care class, report of findings or debate with a detractor.

Receiving

To use the Internet effectively as a receiving tool, start with Google and then learn to construct a systematic investigation and evaluation procedure so you quickly and efficiently get to the information you need. If you want short video tutorials on how to work this technology, you can go to google.com and click on the YouTube icon, or you can go directly to youtube.com—then search for whatever information you're looking for.

Google is so user-friendly that it has itself become the very definition of the service it offers, a verb that means to engage the noun it is identified by. Even if someone might choose another search engine, they still probably say they're googling, as Google has claimed this word in the mind of the marketplace, one reason it is such a powerful brand with unparalleled influence.

For example, at a seminar in London a few years ago, our guest speaker was Dr. Karsten Pedersen, director of one of the largest clinics in the world, based in Sweden, and an expert instructor in Gonstead technique. We had trouble with the compatibility of his PowerPoint with our computers, and in order to make it work, we had to find a way to defeat the security program on our computer.

Sonovagun—my son and producer Jeremy was able to go online, find out specific instructions for exactly our situation, disable the program, and in a few minutes had the problem solved. That's how far-reaching the scope of available information is, billions of pages of data at your fingertips in seconds, and it's increasing at an unprecedented pace. It's mind-boggling.

Google has so many services available, and their leadership in this area is profound and penetrating. It's pretty much futile to try to do it without them, even though the fine print gives them access to your information and the option to do potentially invasive online things with it. The trade-off is mostly worth it.

You're also going to need to choose which communications technologies you wish to include in your strategy, then start to watch, listen, and take in enough online experiences to feel reasonably well-versed so you know the ropes and avoid getting in your own way with clumsy technique and under-informed approaches.

Google, Facebook, Twitter, Instagram, Pinterest, LinkedIn, YouTube, and many other online roads to drive down—no one can master all of them at the same time, so you'll have to decide which ones to study first, and over time you'll be able to coordinate and use them all to their best advantage.

Sending

Receiving information from the web is like drinking off a fire hydrant, and for that reason, when you start to think about and get into position to develop the second big chunk of online utilization, sending, you must understand that you are competing with billions of words by others who feel just as strongly about the importance of their message as you do about yours.

Getting heard is a real art form, and through most of the rest of this chapter we'll be exploring how you can send out your message and get people to respond by becoming and referring new patients, every day.

By learning about the many ways of sending out we'll be exploring, you'll develop mastery at transmitting information, and orchestrating the many options available to you to present your own online personality as you wish.

As a veteran online columnist for over seventeen years, I can tell you I've made most of the mistakes you can make, from just putting my foot in my mouth to inflaming and provoking significant anger and conflict, to inviting harsh feedback, some deserved and some undeserved. I learned from Tony Robbins twenty years ago that the meaning of your communication is the response you get. It's not what you said, or meant to say, or thought you said, it's what the other person gets that counts.

Based on that, I've learned that it all works so much better when we observe some rules and guidelines about how to communicate on the Internet.

Guide To Online Etiquette: reputation.com

As an Internet public service, reputation.com published some basic guidelines to avoid stepping on any online land mines. They recommend using the typical human courtesies, and acknowledge that many have yet to embrace the good manners on the web that they might express more freely in person.

They recommend the "Golden Rule"—to treat others on the web as you would prefer to be treated. They suggest you use your real name rather than a pseudonym of some kind—when your name is associated with a post, it's more likely you will carefully consider the benefits and consequences. This increases both accountability and credibility.

Almost everyone uses the net to search for the histories of job applicants, potential vendors, and customers, and that's why it's so important to keep your online reputation as pristine as you can.

Online reputation management is a vital part of any business marketing you might consider—you want to present yourself in the best possible light at all times.

Web Presence

Who you are on the web is who you are to most of the people who engage you through the web. That means that the benefit of the doubt you may earn with people who actually know you personally typically does not apply when someone's exposure to you is online only.

That means your web presence, your online identity, depends on how well you represent yourself. The artwork, the language, and most importantly, the overall effect of your website and posts will determine who people believe you to be, and while you may believe that you are more than your website, in cyberspace you may not get the chance to prove that.

It's essential that you produce a web presence that is befitting of your status, and consistent with your message. It's hard to do this in a vacuum, so seek coaching, and don't be quick to dismiss feedback you get, even if it isn't articulated kindly—sometimes you get vital information by getting past your upset and being truly objective, hard as that may seem at times.

Remember that whatever you put up on the net will likely stay there in some form forever, even if you try to remove it, so be discriminating, and I suggest you err on the side of caution. Use restraint, especially in putting out edgy materials or anything that could be misinterpreted. Don't be a wimp, but use your best judgment before you send out any communication.

With that said, you want your web presence to be appealing, attractive, and user-friendly. If you are talented at website design, it can be a great manifestation of your creativity, but most will need some advice and/or technical support in getting your site up and running. I suggest you find local professionals to help you, both so you can have someone in striking distance for issues that arise, and also as an opportunity for inter-referral. I'll mention some additional resources along the way.

Logos and catchy names didn't used to mean that much except to huge corporations, since it took so much money to position them in the mind of the marketplace. But with the ease of operation and the modest expense of establishing your web presence, you can get your message and your representative identification symbols out to more people than ever before. The amazing success of Justin Bieber is only one example of an unknown who launched himself on the web and achieved stardom. And as I mentioned before, my weekly column has reached millions of eyes, minds, and hearts—I could never have done that with a traditional print newsletter.

Establishing your web presence depends on your website, your platform or list, your affiliates or strategic alliances, your blog, your use of social media, and your methods of engaging your marketplace.

Search Engine Optimization (SEO)

Throughout this chapter I'll be showing you how I googled topics and came up with writers, bloggers, teachers, and other experts so I could report on the results of my research. It may make you wonder, with all the information out there, why did this data come up instead of something else?

There is a technical term used by online marketers for this phenomenon, known as Search Engine Optimization, or SEO. It's a little complicated, and I can't claim to understand every bit of the technology, but here's the way it basically works.

When you publish something on the net, it's analyzed for its content—sort of like "spiders" crawling over the pages, taking note of which words can be used to make that publication available to those looking for that content. Those words, known as "tags," determine how obvious that page will be—in other words, how close it will be to the top when someone searches for that word.

The closer to the top of the list, the more "hits," in other words, the more people are attracted to click on that particular document. Likewise, the more hits, the closer to the top of the list, so it's a real art to maneuver your website or publication to the top of the list for your industry or type of business.

Google Analytics provides statistics on the number of hits, the frequency of tags, and many other important bits of data you can use to decide what is working and not working in your online communication. Doing this effectively manifests as increased traffic, increased impact, and of course, increased flow of new business. It's very user-friendly—just go to google.com/analytics and it will prompt you from there. Or, as always, you can go to YouTube and search for short video tutorials on this, and pretty much anything else you'd be looking for.

By the way, when you search for a video, the reason the first one you see comes up first is because it had the highest rating among its competitors. That's why you need to become expert in SEO, or hire experts to advise you.

Hunting vs Farming

I want to touch on one more important concept before we dig into some online new patient generating strategies.

I attended and spoke at a marketing seminar conducted by Drs. Patrick and Cynthia Porter, founders of PorterVision, whom many of you know as the developers of the MindFit light and sound technology used to reduce brain stress. They are world class experts in NLP, communication and marketing, and great friends to the chiropractic profession. I'll tell you more about Patrick and Cynthia in Chapter 7 when we talk about back-end fronting, but when I was at this recent program, I heard about the concepts of hunting and farming, an explanation of prospecting for new business that may shine a new light on Internet marketing for you, as it did for me.

I googled "hunting vs farming" and found a concise and well-written article on sitepoint.com, December 5, 2011, written by John Tabitha, called "Hunting or Farming: Which Type of Prospecting is Best?"

He says, "There are two different types of prospecting, and which you choose depends on how hungry you are."

Hunting

You hunt when you're hungry and can't wait for crops to grow. You want food and you want it now. In marketing, hunting takes the form of going out into the marketplace, literally or figuratively, and seeking quick action, a rapid response to your efforts. This provides new business right now, to soothe your hunger.

The problem is, if you are primarily a hunter, you are always on the hunt, because that's how you eat. It's stressful, and there are times you find no prey and go hungry. But you can become skillful at hunting and sustain yourself that way, if you choose.

Farming

When early explorers colonize a new area, they have no choice but to start out as hunters—they haven't had time to cultivate an ongoing source of food so they forage, looking for whatever they can find to eat; wildlife, local plants or whatever.

But astute settlers realize that to create a sustainable lifestyle, it would help if they could predict their food, both by raising crops and herding animals. This is referred to as farming.

So what does this have to do with attracting chiropractic patients?

The settlers had nothing at the beginning. The first thing they probably did after securing shelter was hunt for food. They couldn't plant vegetables and wait until spring before having their first meal. Yet, that's what many new businesses (and practices) do—they wait for people to respond to their ads on social media, and they starve before their marketing has a chance to work.

So how hungry are you? Early settlers needed to make a kill immediately in order to survive. If you're just starting out, you need to do the same. And further, if you find yourself in a lull for whatever reason, you need to get in gear and go slay a beast or two.

The Prehistoric Family

If you were a caveperson in prehistoric times, you might find yourself looking across your dinner table at the hollow eyes and drawn cheeks of your family—they need food, and it falls to you to go find some.

So you go out into the wilderness to find a beast to slay. When do you go home?

When you've slain a beast. There's no point in going home before that—you'd only have to go out again, since your family would still be there, starving.

So your level of focus and commitment must be there for you to make this work.

Notice, farming isn't any easier—you'd have to plow the fields, plant the seeds, water and feed the plants, ward off insects and weather and poachers and who knows what else.

Early citizens learned that a proper blend of hunting and farming is the best way to go. And chiropractors realize the same thing—strategies like public speaking, screenings, and asking for referrals work well as hunting techniques for when you want a quick boost to your new patient flow, whereas health care classes, patient appreciation promotions, networking with professionals, and a strong back end will develop the longer-term relationships that can be farmed over time.

Notice that both are easily done with Internet marketing—you can mail offers to your list for a quick response, or you can send abundant free content to establish a loyal followership, who can then be solicited for repeat business and for new referrals.

Creating the Optimal Blend

Each marketing or advertising method has inherent strengths and weaknesses. Unfortunately, many business owners are looking for the "silver bullet"—the one method that will bring in all the business they need. The reality is that effective marketing is a blend of several or many approaches.

In his "Hunting vs Farming" article, John Tabitha writes:

> Consistently having conversations with people in your target market is the first step. How are you going to get in front of enough of them? Here's where the either-or fallacy hurts most freelancers: either inbound marketing is best, or outbound marketing is best.
>
> (Inbound marketing is advertising with free or very inexpensive content like blogs, video, eNewsletters, social media and search engine optimization that attract people into relationships that lead to sales. Outbound marketing is telemarketing, direct mail, radio and TV, and traditional advertising, designed to go out and get business.)
>
> But you can generate plenty of conversations using both cold-calling and social media. The former is hunting, the latter is farming. Cold-calling is more likely to generate a new client immediately; social media less so. Social media is farming—it takes time for the relationship to flourish, but once it does, the prospect is more likely to hire you because of it.
>
> Just like those early settlers, your marketing goal ought to be to gradually wean yourself away from depending on hunting and into more consistent farming, using hunting as needed or to attract a certain type of patient you desire.

As your crops begin to grow and you begin to domesticate some wild prospects, you'll have a barn full to which to market.

I think this article says it clearly—you must create an appropriate blend of aggressive outreach and cultivation of long-nurtured relationships. This art of shaping your marketing is instrumental in creating fulfillment based on your identity, your vision, and your purpose.

Well, we've talked about a lot of theory so far—now let's roll up our sleeves and get to some ways to attract new patients every day through the Internet.

Using YouTube

You can post your videos, or videos of your choosing, on the net by starting a YouTube channel. It's easy, free, and provides an instant method for you to get your message out. People love videos, and you can quickly learn to produce little videos that will communicate clearly with your audience. Believe it or not, much of what you see on YouTube was recorded with an iPhone or some other relatively low-tech approach.

One of the best examples of effective chiropractic online marketing I know is Dr. Anna Saylor of the Van Every Chiropractic Center of Royal Oak, Michigan. You can find her at VanEveryChiropractic.com, and it's worth your while to check out her web presence.

Go to her website and see how she orchestrates many of the online options—for example, you can click on the YouTube button, and it will take you to her YouTube channel, where she has many videos, most of which are simply case studies or candid snapshots of daily office activities, her technique, or her remarks about some relevant topic.

She has millions of hits, and attracts about fifty new patients a month while she's raising the consciousness of her community and beyond.

And if you'd like to hear a terrific teleclass where Dr. Bob Hoffman interviews Dr. Saylor about her own specific online strategies that have filled her busy practice with high-quality patients, download the free Masters Circle app at either the Apple or Android store, click on the Teleseries button, and scroll down to the class entitled "The Social Media Checklist."

You can start your own YouTube channel and stock it with videos you like (get permission where appropriate), as well as your own videos you can easily learn to record. To open a commercial YouTube channel, just follow these simple steps.

1. Sign in to YouTube at www.youtube.com.

2. Click on All my channels.

3. If you want to make a YouTube channel for a Google+ page that you manage, you can choose it here. Otherwise, click Create a new channel.

4. Fill out the details to create your new channel.

Many people begin their video channels with nothing more than an iPhone, though when I record my video blogs I use a flip cam and a teleprompter app my son and producer Jeremy found for me, called dvprompter—I downloaded it into my iPad and now I can read a scrolling script; cool and fairly easy to use after a short learning curve.

You may even have heard about the webinar version of this book, "The New Patients Every Day Boot Camp" from the three-minute video ad I recorded, which was e-mailed to my platform, posted on social media sites, and put up on our app, website, blog, and YouTube channel. You can easily learn to create and multi-purpose your materials the same way.

Let's shift our attention for the moment from video to the printed word.

eNewsletters and Blogging

As I mentioned, I've been sending out my eNewsletter every week since September of 1997, and it is both a creative outlet and an opportunity to serve regular customers and new business alike.

These days, you hear many Internet advisors suggesting a blog. What's a blog, and how is it different from a newsletter?

I found the answer from certified online consultant Sarah Santacroce on her website simplicityadmins.ch.

> A blog is your hub. On a blog, which ideally is part of your website, you create content, share your knowledge, opinion and experience. Depending on your schedule, you submit monthly, weekly or daily blog posts. These posts are then public, on the Internet, visible to everybody who visits your website, who's subscribed to your feed or who you've shared the post with on Social Media platforms.

> Your blog is also one of the best ways to get more subscribers for your newsletters. They are reading your content, and at the bottom of the blog post you ask them if they'd like to receive regular updates from you via your newsletter.

> A newsletter is a regular communication between you and your subscribers. It is content that's being sent out via e-mail. It may include links to your blog posts, to other content on the Internet, as well as other valuable information for the subscriber. And of course you will also include

occasional promotions, information about workshops you're running or other deals.

You can also send your blog posts as newsletters. Most auto-responder services, like AWeber or MailChimp, for example, have a service to e-mail your blog to your list, but you probably don't want to send the whole thing—remember, one of the main points of having a blog is to bring traffic to your website. Mail them a synopsis or an excerpt that is compelling, with a link to bring them back to your home turf.

If you want to launch a blog, you can simply go to wordpress.com and they will prompt you through the process. Or, if you have a website support and/or marketing company, they can advise you on setting up a blog and coordinating it with the rest of your web presence. The company I use is invigo.ca, led by Bob Mangat—they are immensely creative, and they aggressively pursue the cutting edge of Internet marketing, a characteristic I require in those I work with. This online world moves quickly, and you must be nimble enough to keep up, or work with people who are.

Webinars

One of my key Internet coaches is Brian Edmondson, brian@ Internetincomecoach.com, a super-bright and savvy young marketer who is expert in all aspects of Internet communication. I tap into him in a variety of areas, and there's no better place to start than to share one of the most powerful and untapped ways to reach people and bring in new patients every day—webinars.

When you schedule a talk in your town, and speak to ten or twenty or fifty or two hundred people, you are doing a wonderful service for those people in attendance and the ripples caused by their new understanding.

But what if you could capture your talk and repurpose it, not only for those who experience it when you record it, but from then on, as part of your library of influential information, performed and provided by you?

Using video to memorialize your contribution to the body of knowledge has never been easier, based on the simplicity and transparency of video recording technology—I mean, you can do it on your phone!

But with a short and reasonable learning curve you can present a webinar, with your audio over a PowerPoint, or even a live shoot where you do your presentation on camera, both to broadcast it and also to record it for future use.

Companies like GoToWebinar are set up to support you in these endeavors; they can support up to 1,000 participants, which should more than handle most typical needs for a chiropractic practice. In fact, the original boot camp version of this book was recorded on GoToWebinar, and they did a good job. But then I got a compelling and persuasive letter from Brian, which alerted me to another, newer technology for this service. It's a great example of an e-mail marketing letter, which I share with you with his permission.

Like a "play within a play," you may be moved to participate in this webinar process yourself, but even if not, you can see how someone who wanted to embrace this technology could reach large numbers of potential chiropractic patients for very little money and a reasonable investment in time and energy.

Here's Brian's letter:

> One of the most common questions I get is, "Brian, how can I utilize the power of webinars in my business?

And it's a great question to ask...

You see, one of the best profit-producing promotional strategies that you can use in your business is a live webinar.

But running a successful live webinar that puts money in your bank account requires following a proven, 4-phase blueprint.

Today, I'm going to share with you the first of those phases, and that's Preparation.

Now this isn't how you prepare your content (you're the expert on that one) or even your sales message (that's a topic for another e-mail training series)... but the mechanics and marketing of running the live webinar itself.

In the preparation phase you will decide how you want your content presented.

Depending on the webinar service you use, you may be able to run pre-recorded videos, PowerPoint or Keynote presentations, share your computer screen or even show yourself on a webcam.

The best format you can do is to start with a webcam view so your audience gets to see you, then after your introduction, switch to slides for your content presentation.

Consider which medium works best for your message though, as some niches respond much differently than others.

When it comes to the mechanics of presenting a live webinar to a mass audience, the clear winner is Google Hangout On Air.

Unlike other unreliable webinar services that cost upwards of $500 a month and are limited, Hangouts are backed by Google and YouTube, so you don't need to worry about servers crashing and recordings failing. And best of all—they are free!

However, for marketers there are some serious problems with Hangouts. One of the biggest downsides is that you're limited to just 10 participants. Of course, others can watch your stream, but there's no way of interacting with them, making it difficult to run Q&A sessions, polls, or any kind of group chat. And forget about sharing a link with them to purchase anything.

Of course, this sort of interaction and active participation significantly boosts sales conversions and so is an absolute must. That's why many reluctantly pay the ridiculous prices and suffer through the lousy technology of other webinar software.

Well, that was, until now.

Thanks to my good friends Andy Jenkins and Mike Filsame, who've created software that takes the powerful marketing tools present in other webinar software and applied it to Google Hangouts.

All of the marketing power, but more affordable than you might imagine, considering Google Hangouts do all the heavy lifting for you. Check it out here.

Once you've prepared your content and the platform you're using for your webinar, the next phase is Promotion; but I'll get to that in tomorrow's e-mail training.

- Brian

PS. When choosing webinar software, consider the one created by the giants of the industry - the world's most reliable webinar platform (Google Hangouts) with the most powerful marketing features... created by Andy and Mike.

Edmo Publishing LLC, 922 South Woodbourne Rd., PMB 303, Levittown, PA 19057, USA   Unsubscribe | Change Subscriber Options

This is a beautifully written example of an affiliate promotion, Brian co-venturing with a company called WebinarJam, now commanding a significant market share. (In fact, when I participated in one of his webinars, I saw that Ed Osburn, founder and moderator of the podcast series "The Chiropractic Philanthropist," whom you'll learn more about at the end of this chapter, uses WebinarJam.) Brian is a master at this form of marketing—notice how he is brief and to the point, and gives you valuable, free content. Then, he makes a persuasive offer, and teases you with a cliffhanger about the next bit of content so you are more likely to open the next e-mail from him. Even if you're not ready to buy, you're curious about the next piece of the puzzle.

In this way, he develops a relationship with you, and increases your comfort level about future engagement and sales. Also, he tells you the benefits of his offer, but you have to click to find out the details. In this way you enter his funnel, the pathway toward sales.

I do recommend Brian's coaching, as he has been invaluable to me, not only because of his clear and innovative style, but also his passion to remain up-to-date in the field of Internet marketing. I consider him part of my team. If you speak to him, tell him I said hi.

Designing Your Webinar

Webinars are creative events—they start someplace, go someplace, and end someplace. Boot camps like New Patients Every Day are more focused on education than on sales (though I did mention about a dozen products and services along the way), but you can easily design and offer webinars to chiropractic patients and candidates for care, especially interactive webinars that really engage people. You can serve and educate your current clientele, and create a steady stream of prospective chiropractic patients for you to enroll in your program of care.

Let's talk a little about putting together a webinar. When you approach your first planning session, get into a resourceful state; do some breathing or affirmation or visualization, or move your body in a powerful way, or just think about times you were creative and bright and effective.

Once you're in a resourceful, creative state, focus on developing outcome clarity—what is it that you are aiming to accomplish? Stephen Covey said to begin with the end in mind—what is it that you want to happen?

Once you have outcome clarity, it isn't a bad idea to visualize and affirm your outcome as part of the process. I always include this kind of inner preparation before I launch into any strategy—it makes me more acutely sensitive to details I can use, and I believe it enhances the manifestation of my goals to concentrate my creative power this way. Try it for yourself and see if it seems the same to you.

Now that you have managed your state, chosen your objective, and invoked the higher powers, it's time for the nuts and bolts of planning your webinar. I use a system I call "the creative strategy," which works like this.

The Creative Strategy

Divide your page into a left and right half with a vertical line. On the left side, draw a large rectangle, and divide it into three sections, smaller ones at the top and bottom and a larger one in the middle. These three sections represent the opening of your webinar, the body of your webinar, and the closing of your webinar.

The opening usually has some introductory remarks, maybe some credentialing, but most importantly a story or basic premise that draws people in so they engage and want to continue.

The body is where you present your material, the information you wish to convey or share.

The closing is where you complete your presentation, and make whatever offer you have planned to support the outcome you'd like to accomplish. If it's to get people to come to your office as new patients, then there should be some kind of offer or closing that compels people to take action. You can apply some of the closing techniques you learned in Chapters 2, 3, and 4.

Use the right-hand side of the page to collect copy points, and after you brainstorm out the ideas for your webinar, insert them into the appropriate box, or just draw arrows if you like. This gives you an outline of the complete webinar on one page.

Now, you can write a script and read off a teleprompter or you can free wheel it, depending on your lust for spontaneity and your tolerance for imperfection. But webinars generally benefit from some type of visual—otherwise, it's a teleclass. You can design a PowerPoint, use a webcam to do a live shoot, or record some video segments and intersperse them among your live or PowerPoint segments.

Be creative—while you are competing with some of the very best out there, no one has your message, your style, or your personal charisma. Get your word out so people can experience you, and some will choose you. The idea is to get as many people as possible to consider you, and work at improving the percentage that decide to engage you.

Building Your Platform/List

Whether you use YouTube, eNewsletters, blogs and websites, and/or webinars, you're going to need people to market to, and in online language, accumulating a list of e-mail addresses of people who may be interested in your services is referred to as building your platform. Sometimes the word *platform* is also used to describe the social media vehicles themselves, for example, Facebook or Twitter can be referred to as a platform, so I'll avoid confusion by only using this word to describe your mailing list. But if you hear it used the other way in common usage, you'll be able to figure out what the person is talking about from the context.

For inbound marketing, where you expect people to find you and capitalize on their discovery, you want to maintain a classy and impressive web presence so when people find you, they like what they see. For outbound marketing, you want to learn to skillfully operate and manage your outreach, capitalizing on opportunities with dignity and professionalism.

For those situations that call for sending out a newsletter, video, or sales offer, you want to send to people who are likely to respond. Some online marketers recommend that you continue to e-mail people until they buy or die, but you can maximize the efficiency of your outbound marketing by getting people to opt in, instead of just spamming them. Spam is Internet slang for unrequested and usually unwanted communications that clog up the inbox and pollute the cyber-circuitry. Like junk mail, it is mostly clutter, with occasionally worthwhile information. You are better off transcending spam by getting people to agree to receive your materials by opting in.

I took an outstanding four-module webinar course from Brian last year, and one of the topics he explored in detail was how to build your platform. With his permission, I share a few of these ideas with you.

I think it's apparent that anyone you come across whom you want to include in your work, you'd want to add their address to your list. The problem is, that tends to generate a partially committed customer list, since they are receiving information they may not have asked for or recognize as yours, or is even relevant at all. For this reason you want to get people to come to your website and perform a vital function in online marketing—you want them to opt in.

Opting in means they have gone to your website, landing page, or squeeze page, which is like a sub-website dedicated to a particular project or function, and put in their contact information, often to receive some free content, which opens the door for you to send them more communication.

To get people to opt in, you need to drive traffic to your website, which you can do in many ways. You can use traditional ads, like print media, radio, TV, or direct mail to funnel people toward your website. You can use social media vehicles, like Facebook, Twitter, LinkedIn, and others to spread your address around with some free content, and include links that drive people to your website.

You can also use what Brian refers to as integration marketing. You see, your prospects are already going to certain websites, publications, blogs, and counselors—do some research to discover where your best potential clients visit, and establish a presence there.

For example, you probably already receive e-mails from assorted chiropractic blogs. You could read them, follow some conversations, and when you have something valuable to add, offer it. Be patient. Don't overstate your case; ease into it without holding anything important back. You'll gain a reputation, and others on those blogs who agree with your point of view will refer patients in your area. The Internet connects people who are hundreds or thousands of miles apart, so these are doctors you might not otherwise get to know.

Then, those patients and their referrals become part of your platform. And you can build a database of doctors as an inter-referral network, or to enter into co-ventures as affiliates of products and services you already use that you could share with them. You could market a seminar on your area of expertise to those doctors, or pool resources with them about marketing and patient education ideas. There are layers of profit all over this type of relationship building.

Or, you can go to patient-oriented blogs on nutrition, family health care, pediatrics, chronic pain, or special interest of your choice, and after listening, watching, and reading for long enough, start to make comments, add your two cents and establish a presence there, voicing relevant opinions without overt selling or hyperbole.

It is sometimes permissible to leave a contact address of some sort in your post, so if this is legitimate, it provides a way for people to respond both on the blog and directly to you.

Always observe the etiquette of the particular blog—some are geared toward more exchange, some have slightly different ethics, so learn the ropes before you get tangled up in them.

So, to summarize and simplify this process:

1. Identify top experts in your market.

2. Determine how to integrate with them.

3. Decide what types of content to create.

4. Develop your own content schedule.

5. Master a traffic method and apply it.

6. Dedicate time each week for traffic research.

If you're curious about some of the latest thinking on online marketing strategies, read The Invisible Selling Machine by Ryan Diess. He spells out his methods for reaching and inspiring his list to take action on his offers, something you can instantly adapt to attracting new patients every day.

Twitter

Twitter is a social media giant which allows people to communicate in short language bites, 140 characters at a time. The point of using Twitter, either to follow someone else's posts or offer your own, is to build relationships. It's easy to use it to cross-promote to create direct sales, but for chiropractors, you can recruit followers who are interested in tweets on health and wellness, or you can communicate with other chiropractors all over the world to manifest a dense inter-referral network that can bring in new patients every day.

Construct your Twitter profile to be broad enough to include as many people who may be interested in your tweets as possible. Then, you want to follow those inside your target market, as well as related professionals and areas of interest—you want to know who else is influencing the people you'd like to influence, and what moves them. It may not be what you think, and that's why it's so important to follow before you jump in like a hero and start tweeting. There's a finesse and a set of standards and guidelines you will quickly observe and learn, but it's bad practice to violate them.

You want dialogue with Twitter, not just a one-sided spew of your ideas. Industry experts recommend that you plan about 80% of your tweets in response to others' conversations and 20% that you originate. Your tweets should be relevant to your identity and web presence, and it's good practice to avoid unnecessary controversy or divisive commentary unless you have a specific agenda for doing so. Remember that once you put it out there, you won't be able to retrieve it, as many high-profile celebrities have discovered—just a word to the wise.

You can generate several or many lists that perform different functions for you. There's a program known as TweetDeck that is designed to help you organize your lists.

When you're getting started, commit to ten or fifteen minutes a day for a month or so to follow some key individuals who are putting out messages that help you learn the basics.

When you start to respond and tweet back, you can include links to articles, blogs, remarks on current events, and compliments on others' work. Offering positive feedback on brands makes them interested in you, because once you put it out there, it's searchable and visible to anyone who knows how to look.

Keep it real—veterans will easily pick out the rookies and phonies, so don't try to be something you're not. It's okay to show some vulnerability or inexperience, it makes you more authentic; just don't overstate your case, as always. This elevates the relationship, and earns you the right to be more aggressive when the relationship can handle it.

To get people to notice you, put buttons on your website, use banners, or ask people to trade links and contact information. When you engage people, invite them to follow, like, or participate.

You can click on (or originate) specific conversations, known as hashtags and signified by the number or pound sign, which directs your attention and your responses specifically to that conversation. Also, be careful about outsourcing—it's more about developing the relationship than just marketing, which is why this approach is more about farming than hunting. You can use experts as a resource, but keep your energy and emotions engaged.

Some say that Twitter is used more for connecting with influencers, where Facebook is more for connecting with current and potential customers, though either can be used for both.

Facebook

Facebook is like a giant switchboard, connecting people across the globe minute by minute. It's a smorgasbord of content, and an invitation to spend all your time on trivial stuff. but used effectively, it is one of the most potent of all communications devices.

One of the first rules when entering into a Facebook experience is to decide up front to use your time strategically and efficiently. The pull of Facebook is so strong, and the scope is so immense, many of us who have engaged it have found ourselves following links into uncharted territory, finding more and more compelling reasons to stay on indefinitely and often with marginal ultimate value other than entertainment or pure information gathering.

Some Facebook posts are about eating a bagel, getting caught in traffic or waking up early to a quiet house, and while that may seem important at the time, you will inspire less traffic if you don't remember two things—firstly, other people think their posts are valuable, whether you do or not, so manage your responses to be civil, relevant, and useful. Secondly, if you are going to post something, remember that all those on that list will receive it, and you want it to be worthwhile for them to visit your page and develop their relationship with you.

You should consider both a personal page and a fan or company page, to begin structuring your communications to accomplish more. You will want to like people's posts and respond to them to continue the conversations you find appropriate for you to participate in and build the relationship. You can use this approach to service accounts, meet new friends and influencers, and manage communication.

Facebook users tend to enjoy images, questions, and videos more than just information or commentary, unless the relationship is already highly developed. You can have patients, patients' family and friends, and other neighborhood professionals participate, but always remember that everyone on that list will see those posts so make them kind, practical, and inoffensive. You can share relevant news, but on a list you are using to reach patients and potential patients, my opinion is that it's better to avoid serious controversy that could be misinterpreted or taken out of context.

Again, put in your due diligence to get the hang of it before you bravely put your name on something you broadcast into cyberspace—once you put it out, it isn't that easy to get it back.

There are many Social Media Options

There are many other ways to engage people and develop relationships—Instagram is a popular social network application where you can upload, edit, and caption photos. LinkedIn is designed to network with professionals, while Pinterest is about posting photos, pictures, and graphics in categories, and is also great for promoting practice-related and health and wellness-related topics. If you are planning to coordinate several social media vehicles, consider HootSuite to create the connections between them so when you post on one, your post appears on the others, too—just be careful to manage your lists effectively to prevent sending the right info to the wrong people.

There's a lot more we could talk about here, but you get the idea. This takes a while to learn and master, but there are plenty of ways to generate new patients every day by applying these ideas and this amazing technology.

Learning to use systematic e-marketing can streamline your marketing process and save considerable money from direct mail, print advertising, and other more standard approaches. It's not that these are bad, but e-marketing reaches deeply into a demographic that may not even be aware of the more typical methods. It's worth your while to learn the rules, so here are a few fundamentals to get you started.

Your best traffic is your own e-mail list—once people opt-in, create a welcome series of e-mails to guide them through the preliminary decision-making that leads them to starting the new patient process. This is how you convert online prospects to new patients.

You want to provide free content at first, but you can invite people to consider becoming new patients by making an offer. Generally, newcomers to this methodology may be too heavy-handed or too timid, but it is acceptable to use a ratio of one-to-one on free content and making an offer, or as much as three letters with free content for each offer.

The content can be a short passage, 500-1,000 words at most, or even better, an audio or video that adds value and makes the person glad he or she received it. That buys you the latitude to pitch them on chiropractic care, nutritional advice, personal training, wellness programs, and a host of other relevant services and products you offer. Aim for at least once a week if not twice a week or more, plus a monthly recap to keep people engaged.

If you use audio or video, keep it concise—as a rule of thumb, each 150-175 words of copy is about a minute of audio or video, so you can plan accordingly. I tend to click on short posts, and I often don't get to the longer ones even if I save them—generally, you wouldn't expect something from your prospects or patients that you wouldn't do yourself.

Don't just promote, add value. And make it personal, so people connect—this too is about building relationships, and you are probably recognizing a theme here—this is more about pulling than pushing.

Deliver what you promise, and once people buy, segment your list to make the content and offers even more precise and useful for those people. You can use date-limited e-coupons or certificates to drive home your offer, and also to manage the influx of people and track where they may have come from, which builds your statistics to interpret your results and plan future promotions.

Once people opt in, your basic format for follow-up looks something like this:

1. Create your own welcome e-mails.

2. Develop your conversion follow-up series.

3. Determine your follow-up schedule.

4. Continue to add follow-up e-mails to your auto-responder.

5. Commit to sending frequent content and offers.

So, you can see that throughout this chapter, I accessed many of the online basic services I've been talking about—I googled the information of absolute strangers and found exactly what I was looking for, for the price of mentioning their names and contact information so you can find them, engage them, exchange with them, and profit from each other in ways that may not be immediately obvious. And, I used YouTube tutorials to verify or complete much of the information I shared here.

Some of these techniques are farming, and some are hunting. You can get a quick influx of new patients with webinars, search engine optimization, date-limited e-coupons or certificates, fliers, or other solicitations.

Or, you can establish relationships with people and build your platform, using social media, sending drip e-mail, newsletters, or attracting them to your blog or website, so over time they see the value of becoming your client or customer. YouTube videos are flexible and can be used in both hunting and farming.

Obviously, both hunting and farming are necessary, so please understand that hunting can bring in new patients every day, and farming can bring in new patients every day, over time. Depending on your current circumstances, only you can determine the appropriate ratio.

Podcasts

One of the best ways to engage your prospects and patients is to supply them with a steady stream of relevant, practical content, and if you can do it for free, you have a winning formula that can attract all the new people you could possibly handle. A great way to do this is to establish a podcast program, a modern way to distribute your content that is easy, inexpensive, and penetrates deeply into your potential audience.

The major proponent of podcasting in chiropractic is Dr. Ed Osburn, founder and moderator of The Chiropractic Philanthropist (dred@thechiropracticphilanthropist.com). Dr. Ed brings some of the top thinkers and entrepreneurs in chiropractic to his listeners, and also offers courses and training on how you can use podcasts to reach a bigger audience and attract more new people into your practice.

I recommend that you subscribe to The Chiropractic Philanthropist and The Masters Circle podcasts—you'll get tons of free content about all aspects of chiropractic practice, for free, delivered to your phone or device with no effort on your part. All you do is listen. And once you see how powerful this method of communication can be, you'll be tempted to use it yourself. Take Dr. Ed's training, or google how to create a podcast—after a short learning curve, you can use this technique to spread your message far and wide. For many doctors, this may be all that is required to bring in new patients every day.

While it wasn't possible to cover every detail, I've provided you with many resources to further your studies in this ever-expanding field of Internet marketing and information distribution.

Now the fun begins—you get to prepare your artist's palette, shaping your web presence and your online strategies to support your optimal blend of hunting and farming to generate the new patient flow you want.

Points to Remember

1. Modern marketers familiarize themselves with the many online methods of promoting their message and their practice. Your web presence determines how people perceive you, so observe proper online etiquette, and use the various online options wisely.

2. When you are very hungry for new patients, you'll have to develop hunting techniques. When you want to develop longer-term relationships with people to engage them more deeply, you'll have to develop farming techniques.

3. Tap into the expertise of coaches, advisors, and companies that can save you time, energy, and money.

Actions to Take

1. Dedicate some time to design an online strategy, first to gather, systematize, and store relevant information, then to prepare and send out content that can initiate and develop a relationship with your prospective audience.

2. Pick one or two online options and focus your attention on them to learn how they might work to engage potential new patients.

Questions to Ponder

1. Imagine which online options will work better for you in hunting, and which will work better for you in farming.

2. Which experts would streamline your path toward online mastery?

This concludes Chapter 6, introducing you to Internet marketing. In Chapter 7, called "Back-End Fronting," we'll be discussing an innovative way to use all the different services and products you offer to attract new patients every day.

CHAPTER 7
Back-End Fronting

Back-End Fronting is a term I made up to describe a marketing and new patient attraction process I discovered early in practice.

Two Common Denominators

As a student, I observed that the chiropractors who seemed to be most successful, both clinically and financially, had two distinct qualities in common. Firstly, they had certainty about chiropractic and their role in the healing process. Secondly, they found a way to move the patient emotionally, beyond just the information they conveyed. Some did it with motivation, some with leadership, still others with fear, but it became clear to me that if I was going to be successful, I had to learn from the experiences of those who came before, and this distilled wisdom turned out to shape my ten years in practice.

My First Outcome

You see, by the time I graduated chiropractic college in December of 1977, I'd had a successful clinical tour, and was very comfortable taking care of people. My understanding of the two qualities I had recognized in my role models had evolved, and as I launched into practice, I had two outcomes for every office visit. First, I was determined that no one would come into my office with a subluxation complex I couldn't figure out. This was my way of developing certainty.

I already had complete confidence in Innate Intelligence, and I accepted that the limiting factor was my own ability to solve the patient's riddle, to interpret the body's wishes and convert on them, delivering just what was called for, no more, no less.

I needed to become a master of the art of chiropractic—that's how I would gain the certainty I knew I needed to satisfy this first outcome.

So, I embarked upon a ten-year quest for the best techniques to locate and correct nerve interference. My enthusiasm led me down the technique rabbit hole.

Down the Technique Rabbit Hole

My earliest influences in chiropractic helped to shape the technique of my first years in practice. I had learned upper cervical technique, classical Palmer style HIO from Dr. Thomas LeRoy Whitehorne, may he rest in peace; a tall, thin chiropractic warrior with gleaming blue eyes and a shock of white hair. Dr. Whitehorne ran the BJ Palmer Clinic in the late fifties and early sixties, before he came back to Brooklyn, New York, to practice and teach philosophy and technique at my alma mater, New York Chiropractic College, originally the Columbia Institute of Chiropractic.

We used to go to Whitehorne's office on Wednesday nights and he would adjust us and show us cool stuff he had from his heyday at Palmer, sharing many stories of chiropractic miracles and the importance of keeping Innate in chiropractic practice. I was blessed to learn from him.

Midway through chiropractic college, Whitehorne had introduced me to Pierce-Stillwagon Technique, a derivative of Thompson Terminal Point, using drop pieces on the table that are still popular today. I loved the HIO adjustment because of the intensity of the dynamic thrust, and now I could get the same kind of dynamism adjusting other areas besides the atlas.

Soon thereafter, I became intrigued with Applied Kinesiology (Dr. George Goodheart) and Sacro-Occipital Technique (Dr. Major DeJarnette), AK and SOT, and I took a lot of courses in advanced technique. I was still validating myself and gaining certainty, because I wouldn't stand for anyone walking into my office with a subluxation complex I couldn't figure out.

I loved AK because it gave me a hands-on method of asking the body what it wanted. I was accustomed to using a nervo-scope with my upper cervical work, and a derma-thermograph for the Pierce-Stillwagon, an ancestor of the Pro-Adjuster concept. Many don't realize that it was Vern Pierce who inspired the early research on the Pro-Adjuster.

But I wasn't satisfied that I was really on target with my technique until I found Directional Non-Force technique, DNFT, the brainchild of Dr. Richard Van Rumpt, who came from the lineage of SOT, but branched off as he created his own technique.

Part of the DNFT analysis was the short leg reflex, an evolution of the AK muscle testing method known as therapy localization, where the doctor challenges an area and tests a muscle to determine if that area is in alignment or needing correction.

With Van Rumpt's short leg reflex, you could physically challenge the area, test the leg length, and see if one leg got short. With a little experience, this turns out to be an extremely efficient and high percentage way to interrogate the body and identify the appropriate intervention points.

Dr. Tedd Koren credits DNFT as part of the inspiration for his Koren Specific Technique, along with Dr. Lowell Ward's stressology.

In fact, when you've done this for a while, the physical touches become symbolic, and an experienced DNFTer can question the body by visualizing the affected parts and deriving a strategy from the vibrational connection.

Word got around that I was getting results most chiropractors were not achieving, and other DCs started to send me patients; a great way to get new patients every day, just have other local chiropractors send you their problem cases.

I had studied AK and SOT with Ken Davis, whom I'll talk about a little later when we discuss Natural Force Healing. Ken and another friend and mentor, Jerry Greenberg, were studying the work of M. L. Rees, who had evolved his concepts of cranial work and soft tissue orthopedics into an ultra-modern approach known as harmonics.

Harmonics was the culmination of a brilliant mind working at solving the riddle of vibrational healing—Rees, who had a background in electronics engineering, discovered that he could influence patients at the cellular level by introducing micro-vibration generated by crystalline piezoelectric devices he invented and built.

This was later in my career, and I finally figured out that I could market myself to different groups based on my diversity when I started studying harmonics.

I had heard of a New Age type of group (remember, this was the mid-eighties), who were into crystal healing and vibrational techniques, so I asked them if they'd be interested in hearing about my work with harmonics.

They jumped at the chance, and that created a warm relationship that yielded many happy patients and many stimulating conversations. Many of those people became great chiropractic patients, too—but more about that later.

I saw amazing results with this vast array of techniques. But you may be wondering, why have I told you about my technique odyssey, when I should be helping you attract new patients every day?

I confess this was one of my greatest shortcomings in practice—the failure to capitalize properly on the tremendous back end I had developed, without having any policies or procedures for promoting them, charging for them, and creating a more equal exchange between me and those I served. I used to throw all this stuff into a standard office visit, without realizing that there was a completely ethical way to profit, plus an opportunity to market these tools separately and broaden my appeal to a wider spectrum of people.

That is exactly what I want to help you prevent in your practice—missed opportunities on profit and new patients, based on underdeveloped back-end presentation and positioning, both in your office and in the marketplace. The remainder of this chapter will concentrate on that opportunity.

Anthony Robbins and NLP

One more story about practice—in the early eighties, patients started coming into my office telling me about this amazing speaker they had seen, who spoke a mile a minute, had really big teeth, played loud rock and roll, and at the end they all walked on fire. Of course, I'm talking about Anthony Robbins, at the time in his early twenties and about to rise meteorically through the ranks of motivational seminar leaders to emerge as an all-time great.

At first I batted them away—no thank you, I prefer my motivational speakers with smaller teeth—and I saw no particular value to walking on hot coals, so I resisted at first. But there was something about what they were saying.

Then fate stepped in, and the coaching and seminar company of which I was a member, Markson Management, brought him in as a guest speaker.

A few minutes into his presentation, I was hooked—it launched a twenty-five-year crusade where I sought to understand human behavior at the deepest level, where I became one of Tony's top instructors, and gladly supported him in his ascent to fame and global impact.

I became consumed with working above atlas, which ultimately squeezed me out of practice and led me to be here with you today.

The Roots of my Back-End Fronting

But not before it dawned on me that I had a very marketable commodity in my behavioral engineering skills. I began to recruit patients from my practice who wanted to pursue shifts in their behavior, and we got sensational results. This time, though, instead of including it in my standard office visit, I structured separate office hours to do these interventions, and a counseling practice manifested side-by-side with my chiropractic practice.

Some of those counseling clients moved over to the chiropractic side, an early experience with back-end fronting. I'll be showing you how I did that, and how you can do it, so you can use the other things you do in practice besides adjusting to appeal to patients who might need that as a trigger to begin their relationship with you.

I earned my Master Practitioner certificate for neurolinguistic programming, or NLP, and served as a Master Trainer for Tony, and as such, moved up the ranks, first as a practitioner, then as a counselor and eventually as a consultant.

Soon, as a coach for Larry Markson, I had the biggest consulting practice in the country for a non-owner, overseeing more than three hundred offices each month.

From my experiences coaching thousands of chiropractors, it became apparent that I had overlooked many chances to expand my practice and serve more people in more ways. If my foundational techniques were upper cervical, terminal point and full spine diversified, when I started including AK and SOT, that could have been a back end, and I could have promoted primarily on that, attracting a different clientele.

When I discovered DNFT, there were so few people using this astoundingly potent and subtle technique, it was another missed opportunity to promote non-force work as a back end pushed up front.

And surely the harmonics work, where under my care a blind lady regained her sight, numerous tumors went into remission, and many infertile women conceived, and even a carotid artery that didn't need to be stripped after my vascular enhancement sequences, would have been an incredible draw to bring in new people that may or may not have been interested in chiropractic care.

If only I'd realized at that point that each of these services was actually part of my back end, I wouldn't have included all of it in the office visit fee. I want to make sure you don't fall into the same trap, because if you invest in your education, put in the time and effort to become expert at specialized approaches, and put yourself on the line dealing with challenging cases, it's not inappropriate to be compensated properly; not excessively, but fairly.

So let's explore the structure and mechanics of back-end fronting, so you can use it to attract new patients every day.

Back-end fronting is choosing one of your services or products that is not your main service or product and featuring it to attract new business, and also open the possibility of them being interested in your main service as well—but we'll get to that later on, because there is a finesse to doing that correctly. For now, let's look at some examples of basic back-end fronting.

Martial Arts or Yoga

Let's say you are a martial arts or yoga enthusiast, and as you move up the ranks, you begin to take on students of your own. Those students know you as their martial arts or yoga instructor, not their doctor of chiropractic. In fact, many of your students would probably not relate if you tried to pitch them on chiropractic at the studio or dojo, because that's not how they know you and not what they expect of you.

So, it seems out of context to try to sell them a program of chiropractic care when what they are after is martial arts or yoga training.

There is a finesse at converting someone to your main service, and some people may never make that transition. You have to make that okay, and if they become a chiropractic patient, great. If you develop the relationship effectively, many will. But you never want to lure someone in on a pretense—that's called a bait and switch, where you promise one thing and then try to sell another. Today's consumer is never fooled by that.

That's why, ethically, you have to set up your back end front so it can stand alone. There are methods we'll discuss soon that demonstrate how to bridge this gap when appropriate so they can fully engage your services without making them feel misled in any way.

We're going to investigate back-end fronting from a variety of perspectives, featuring such back end favorites as nutrition, massage, personal training, MindFit, advanced chiropractic techniques, and serum thiol testing, all effective services and products that can attract new patients and give you an opportunity to expand your influence by exposing a new audience to your ideas on health and wellness.

Whatever it takes to bring people into your tent, whether they fully utilize your services or only take advantage of a small portion of your scope of practice, they are that much better for it, and you can find ways to maximize their value and your return.

Nutrition

Let's look at a simple back end front, where a DC who uses full spine diversified technique wants to open a new referral pool by choosing a back end item to move up front. Let's say this doctor drinks a Greens First shake every day, as a nutritional supplement and to alkalize the physiology. How can we take this back-end staple and put it up front?

You could put a display in the reception area so that people who accompany your patients ask about it. You could distribute brochures, either in print or online. You could do a talk about alkalizing, or sell books on the negative effects of acidity, perhaps by M. T. Morter or Don Hayes, or the expert of your choice. You could post a selfie while you're enjoying your shake, with a compelling caption, and get a conversation going. You can do a mall show or screening, but instead of spinal checkups, offer questionnaires and spot counseling on alkalizing, likely to recruit people who are interested in a more metabolic approach to health.

These are all methods of generating a relationship with someone new, who might not yet be up to the point of understanding the importance of regular chiropractic care, but does want to engage on some level with a health and wellness advisor. You can step into that role. Usually it's a recommendation you'd make every day anyway, but when you take your back end and put it up front, you reach people who might otherwise have looked past you.

Take the right leadership actions, and it's likely that your relationship with these health care consumers will expand over time. Be patient, earn his or her confidence, and you'll get your chance. For now, serve them in the way that attracted them, so they get more comfortable with you and begin to trust you. Do nothing to disrupt this trust, as it is an important cornerstone of your developing relationship with this person.

Let's say that someone who is in your reception area, waiting for a friend who is in with you, notices a brochure about Greens First and approaches the front desk to ask about it.

Your front desk CA needs to know to direct the prospective customer's attention properly—the very least that is acceptable would be to pleasantly say, "Many of our patients enjoy great results with this product. The doctor prefers to explain how it's used for your best advantage—in just a few minutes I can make that happen. Please have a seat and I'll give you a little more information to look at." Then in the doctor's next break, the CA makes the connection.

The doctor would congratulate the patient on recognizing the opportunity to simply and inexpensively improve his or her health. There are no contraindications I know of to this kind of generalized nutrition, so give the person some background information, some instructions on how to use the product, and make the sale, taking contact information in the transaction.

At the end, suggest that after a week or two of using the product, to call the doctor and check in on how it's going. The doctor should make a note to follow up, to make sure the customer is using the product, to encourage the use if not, and to receive any questions about the person's experience. About three weeks into the program, make a time for the patient to come back, fill out a quick questionnaire on their results, and sell them another can, this time with the "boost" supplemental shake to upgrade the program.

As the relationship develops, ask about other opportunities to enhance nutrition to improve health, starting to broaden the scope of the relationship. Stay within your awareness of the patient's values, so they feel you know them and are making recommendations consistent with what they know they need and want.

When you sense that the connection is strong, you can begin to explain how the proper use of foodstuffs depends on the body being able to process the intake properly, and that these physiological processes are enhanced by chiropractic care. Now you're guiding the person toward a full-scale utilization of your services, back end front, but now fully engaged as a patient using your main services as well as the product that initiated the relationship.

This process can be accelerated or delayed based on your interpretation, but even if you decide to be aggressive and pitch additional products and services on the first encounter, be wise enough to stay within the patient's professed values hierarchy, and you have a better chance of making a deal. Selling to your values instead of the patient's values won't work nearly as well—if you aren't sure, try it and see.

Massage

One of the most popular back-end fronting opportunities is massage, especially bringing chair massage to places of business and mall shows.

If you're considering using massage in your practice, please check the local and state regulations—you may need a license, certain insurances, and you may or may not qualify for third-party payment. It's your responsibility to know your relevant rules structure, so start by making sure it's legitimate for you to use massage.

Massage is becoming one of the most popular services available because it feels really good, and it's really good for you. This makes it an appealing back-end service, because it's a relatively easy sell, with a reasonable profit margin.

It's also easily deliverable without tremendous pomp and circumstance, requiring only the most cursory history and briefest exam—in fact, the application of the massage in many ways serves as the examination, making it among the most streamlined and immediate healing tools you can incorporate.

It also makes it a natural back-end fronting opportunity. If you offer massage in your office, you probably add it to a program of chiropractic care, and rightly so, when it's in the patient's best interest.

There are lots of people out there who can easily rationalize the value of massage, yet they're still far away from seeing how chiropractic could benefit them. I'm not saying this is desirable, I'm just saying it's extremely common. There are people who would be interested in visiting your massage department, and may or may not ever end up in your chiropractic office. Some will, some won't; so what?

Your office becomes a place where they visit and purchase services, upon which you profit, and also their referrals can be massage, chiropractic, or massage and chiropractic clients, all good for them, all good for you.

There are several ways to back end front with massage. You can do a talk on the benefits of massage in your office and have your patients invite guests. Include a demonstration of some sort so they see what massage looks like and get a sense of how compelling it is for them. You'll get some of these guests to come in for a session, perhaps as part of a special deal or package, and then you have the opportunity to impress them and offer them a program of care.

Remember that the finesse of back-end fronting is to avoid the land mine of selling based on your values instead of theirs. They may well want other services you offer, and of course the centerpiece is regular chiropractic care, to reduce stress in the brain, nerve system, and spine.

But if you take the patient toward your outcomes too rapidly, and they perceive that you are jamming their gears by guiding them away from what they thought they signed up for, they feel manipulated, and typically disengage.

So if someone is attracted in because of massage, let them enjoy the program of massage, and spend a little time getting to know them, developing a relationship and eliciting their values. Find out what's in it for them to partake of massage, and only when you fully understand what they get out of massage can you begin to pitch other services and products—but always based on the outcomes they say they want.

Your challenge is to show them how what you do helps them get something they already want, and when you do this elegantly, they respond and reward you by allowing you to serve them at an even deeper level.

When you engage the massage patient, ask what benefits they are realizing through their experience with massage in your office. They may say something like, they feel more relaxed, less stressed, that a body part like their back or neck feels looser and better, and other stuff like that.

Listen carefully, because you're going to use that information to connect the dots for the patient, and help them see how they can do even better when they capitalize on some of the other services and products you offer that take them even higher on that scale of satisfaction.

You might say, "Let me make sure I heard you right—you say massage helps to reduce your stress and relax your back, and makes your body feel limber, do I have that right?" The patient says yes, and you continue, "So if there was something else you could be doing that would make you feel even less stressed, relax your back even more and have it last longer, and help you feel even more flexible, would you want to know about it?" They say yes, and you have framed your chiropractic care in terms of their values, not yours.

Now, don't present chiropractic care the way you would if you were free-forming in front of a group—this patient has told you in ultra-specific personal terms what he or she wants and is already experiencing. If you start gabbing about nerve interference, brainwaves or whatever, even if it seems relevant to you it's distracting for them, and makes them think you don't know what they are interested in.

Keep your early conversation focused on how what you do adds value to them in the ways they have described, and you'll earn the right to expand your service to them, quickly or slowly, but you will most often get the chance to expand it.

That has to be true if you frame your additional service so they can clearly see that it will support those values they have revealed to you. After all, people do what they do for one of two reasons—either because they want to, or because they have to. If you can crack that code in their own language, you can tap into the internal forces that move them toward your services in a truly genuine and proper way, because it is based on how it fits their needs, defined by them.

This is a higher level of back-end fronting—not only to bring in new business based on services and products other than your primary service, but to elicit their values and show them how other services, especially your primary service, can give them even more of what they really want, or even less of what they want to avoid.

MindFit

My favorite back-end fronting product is MindFit, the brainchild of Patrick and Cynthia Porter, PhD psychologists who are experts in language, behavior, and brain function. They have developed a brain-tuning process that uses light and sound to balance your brainwaves, reduce your stress, and influence all aspects of your health. There are programs that support weight reduction, improve sleep, break habits and addictions, and hundreds of others.

I use MindFit regularly, and I believe it is a powerful resource for better health, deeper sleep, enhanced focus, and a list of other benefits. I can't recommend it any more highly.

The implementation is relatively simple—there are dark-lens glasses with lights mounted inside that flash through the patient's closed lids in specific sequences that tune the brain, while they are listening through headphones plugged into a specially programmed iPod, iPad, or other device.

The recordings, with powerful healing words nestled in a backdrop of magical sounds and frequencies, can be offered a la carte or in a series, designed to address a spectrum of problems, as well as supply personal growth and brain wellness technology. It's a direct route to brain-based wellness, and works perfectly with chiropractic to reduce brain and nerve system stress and optimize health expression.

MindFit is a natural for back-end fronting because it operates both as a standalone and also in conjunction with a variety of other products and services. You could pick any series and it will spawn a list of other profit centers.

For example, if you promote a weight reduction program, you can roll in personal training, nutritional counseling, supplements and meal substitutes, private coaching, group workshops, laser treatments—well, you get the idea, lots of profit centers.

Notice, all of these products and services revolve around the patient's primary outcome, which was to work toward a target weight. Yes, I want them to get chiropractic too, and you will, too, but you'll need to find a way, based on their values, to demonstrate the relevance. Until then, don't force the gears and distract them from their outcome—they are paying customers who are buying from you, don't confuse them. If you do a good job with the part of your service they want now, you'll get a chance to explain how your other services fit their needs. Be patient, and let the process unfold.

When you gain trust, you can expand their set of outcomes, but be careful not to undermine the relationship by appearing to up-sell them based on your intentions rather than their best interests. As long as you stick with their priorities, you're on safe ground.

You can use talks to promote MindFit, or mall shows, where setting people up with a sample session attracts new people consistently. Print ads and brochures also work well for MindFit, but test your headlines carefully to expose the benefit of the program you are promoting. Needless to say, engaging people personally and handing out cards is always productive.

Patrick and Cynthia are masters at training on these tools and techniques—their PorterVision programs and products have my highest recommendation.

MindFit is also one of the easiest transitions into chiropractic care and other products and services you offer.

When you market to stress reduction patients, you can explain that there are other ways to reduce stress, including massage and chiropractic, where you combine working on the mind with working on the body.

When you market to weight reduction patients, it's natural to make nutritional recommendations and offer meal substitutes, alkalizing shakes, appetite suppressants and supplements. It's only a little less obvious that if the body is not metabolizing properly due to interference in its control mechanism, some corrective chiropractic care is called for.

With patients who want to sleep better, you can offer mattresses, massage, pillows, and natural relaxants. If you find that they have muscular tension, limited or arrested movement, or evidence of brain imbalances that could preclude sound sleep, then chiropractic care should also be offered.

This is probably bringing up some cross chatter for you, as it did at first for me. After all, we're chiropractors, and we want to sell people chiropractic, because we know it's the best thing for them. But think about how often you tell people about chiropractic, and how often you are rejected or ignored, compared to how often you are embraced—could it be that we are selling based on our values instead of being sensitive to our customer's values?

We talk about freedom from nerve interference, brain balancing, or a healthy spine—but very few people are evolved to the point where they can seek that as their primary interest. Rather, they have means values that lead toward those ends—we need to learn to work with those means values, and back-end fronting is designed to open these new minds and these new referral pools.

These people will buy from you; maybe not everything or even what you consider the most important thing, but they are buying something you sell, ostensibly because you think it's a good service or product. If you build the relationships and satisfy them based on what they are coming in for, you'll get a shot to take your relationship to new levels as you go forward together.

Not everybody will get all the way to the finish line. But many will, and the others are all coming into your establishment, spending money, and making referrals. That can't be bad, and it's fun and productive to work on your tools of engagement and enrollment to coach as many people as possible to take full advantage of your services.

Anyway, I recommend MindFit for your own personal use, and also as an outstanding back-end fronting opportunity that can bring in new patients every day all by itself. It's inexpensive to operate, clinically potent, and very profitable. And when you talk to Drs. Porter, mention that Dennis sent you.

Advanced Chiropractic Techniques

As you heard me talk about before, I used a lot of fancy chiropractic technique, and because I was young and less experienced, I left a lot of money on the table by not charging a premium for advanced techniques that took considerable extra time and expertise and had significant extra value.

Throughout my thirteen years as a student and practitioner, I spent tens of thousands of dollars on technique courses, and modern technique keeps getting better and better. Many of these techniques are perfect for back-end fronting.

Cranial Release Technique

When I was in practice, I enjoyed and became skillful at cranial adjusting. At first I used SOT cranial, Basic One, Basic Two, Reciprocal Tension Membrane Rocker Technique, Fruit Jars and Parietal Lifts . . . what fun. I also used Applied Kinesiology flavored TMJ technique, and used the Temporo-Sphenoidal Line as a diagnostic tool to track organ circuitry as well as spinal distortion.

I was so absorbed in exploring the amazing miracles of human physiology, I forgot that most chiropractors had not invested what I had in my post-graduate education and the hundreds of extra hours of training and working toward clinical mastery. It would have been completely reasonable to use these techniques as a back end front, to attract different clientele other than through general referral, which is how I attracted two-thirds of my patients.

Any of the techniques I'm going to mention are easily adapted to talks, screenings, and mall shows, and advertising of all kinds, to put these specialized approaches up front for people to see and be attracted toward.

These days, when I want cranial adjusting, I go to Dr. Bill Doreste, founder of Cranial Release Technique, CRT (cranialrelease.com). It's a specialized cranial contact that effectuates a full spine adjustment in a minute or two, and it is a powerful asset to have CRT in your toolbox. It's massively potent, highly efficient, extremely gentle, is performed face up or sitting so it's comfortable for any patient, and its exclusivity commands a premium fee.

Extremities Adjusting

Some of you know that in 2006, I was at a Winners Circle event in Park City, Utah, and one of the events was a bicycle ride through the mountains amidst natural splendor that is unparalleled.

I was having a grand time, until I learned why beginners should stay off intermediate trails—I hit a ditch, joined the "endo" club, meaning I went end-over-end over the handlebars, and landed hard on my neck, back, and shoulder.

I was dazed, and as I sat up and came to, one of the other riders said, "Look, his shoulder is dislocated!" I looked down to my right, and my arm was sticking out of my chest. In shock, I reacted without thinking, and reflexively shoved my arm back into its socket. Another member did some shoulder first aid, and I kind of felt okay, until I tried to stand up, and realized I was pretty messed up.

It was off to the ER, and nothing was broken, just dislocated; the humerus out of the glenoid, and the clavicle off the sternum. The MDs had nothing to offer but a sling and some painkillers I didn't take, opting for two Advil, a night's rest, and then back to the seminar. I even taught my class that day.

But I really wasn't okay. I was getting adjusted, but I had pain, and worse than that, it felt like my skeleton just wasn't fitting together right. I asked a dear friend and outstanding chiropractic orthopedist, Scott Surasky, whom he thought I should see, and without hesitation, he said Mitch Mally (mrmally@live.com).

So, I flew out to Las Vegas to catch Dr. Mally, who travels constantly teaching his extreminars, as well as running a thriving practice in Davenport, Iowa. He examined me, and made so much sense—it was the scapula that needed to be adjusted, then the clavicle and the humerus. I remembered that I had fallen directly on my scapula, and wondered why no one else had thought to adjust it. I felt immediate relief, and he adjusted me a few more times that weekend, gave me some rehab exercises, and sent me home.

Through his adjustments and advice, I have regained full use of my shoulder with no surgery; a complete recovery. So needless to say, I am a big fan of Dr. Mally's. He teaches all over. Catch his act; he has an extraordinary mastery of his subject matter, the adjustment of the extremities.

Extremity adjusting is a terrific back-end fronting option. You can do presentations at golf and tennis clubs. Recruit pros at those clubs to refer you patients. Do print or radio advertising for common extremity complaints, or write articles for sports and fitness magazines. You can publish a blog or newsletter, do direct mail or e-marketing, or put up relevant material on social media. Extremity problems are so common, it's easy to attract people for specific conditions—just remember the finesse of converting them to chiropractic patients, based on their values, not yours.

Functional Neurology

The Masters Circle has spearheaded a movement in chiropractic referred to as brain-based wellness. With clinical psychologists Patrick and Cynthia Porter and chiropractor Richard Barwell, Bob Hoffman and I have worked toward helping doctors learn the language of brain stress, a condition that is a lot easier for patients to understand than traditional chiropractic terminology. Consider introducing subluxation consciousness after the patient enrolls—brain stress is a more compelling description of their condition to engage average patients.

If you can, study the work of Dr. Ted Carrick, the premier functional neurologist in chiropractic today. Any of his courses or those taught by his faculty are worth your while.

The interventions offered by functional neurologists may or may not resemble typical chiropractic adjustments, but the intent is to restore nerve system function by rehabilitating the brain. It is, to me, an evolutionary application of chiropractic reasoning, and a natural back end front, as so few doctors can provide this advanced approach. Once the brain rehabilitation is established, many patients will be fine with more standard chiropractic care, and should typically need less care and hold adjustments better.

NeuroInfiniti

Speaking of functional neurology, Dr. Richard Barwell is an intellectual visionary whose NeuroInfiniti instrument provides a method of calibrating brain function and is simple enough to use in any chiropractic office.

By baselining brain stress and measuring the patient's response in terms of brain recovery and rehabilitation rather than symptom remission, the conversation organically shifts away from how we feel and moves toward how we are functioning. This makes the NeuroInfiniti a natural back-end fronting opportunity, since patients who may not think they need a chiropractor would readily admit to having brain stress. Talks, mall shows, networking, and in-office promotions to that effect would all attract such patients, not to mention referrals.

Also, there are bio-feedback and neuro-feedback systems built into the NeuroInfiniti, a simple and productive profit center that can also be pushed up front to attract yet another stripe of new patient.

NRC

Neurologic Relief Centers (nrc.md) offers a specialized technique that has a profound impact on patients who have severe neurological disease. Patients with fibromyalgia, multiple sclerosis, Parkinson's, migraine headaches, Lyme disease, and many others have responded favorably, and the good news is, the testing, which can be done in minutes, is a strong indicator of the effectiveness of the course of care—a test that yields measurable relief usually foretells a positive response to the course of care.

NRC makes no claim to cure these serious conditions, but rather to provide significant relief. The physiological improvements are attributed to reducing meningeal stress, like many cranial approaches, such as Sacro-Occipital Technique and even HIO are designed to do.

But NRC seems to have a "special something extra" for these tough neurological cases, and as such, has developed a business model that can be run outside the usual policies that would typically accompany a chiropractic program of care. They have positioned themselves as a premium technique, and therefore a premium fee is commanded.

If you market to these patients, many of whom are expert in the available options and why they don't work, you will find a clientele who are motivated and discerning—and when you help them, they tell their friends, because they tend to participate in support groups, to connect with people who can relate to what they have to deal with. Help one of these patients, and you'll get a bunch more to help.

Putting a specialty technique like NRC out front, instead of marketing your more typical chiropractic services, broadens your appeal to an audience that might have otherwise overlooked you. These patients are looking for something specific, and if you seem like it, they will be attracted where they might not have felt the same about your mainstream style of practice.

In this way, by putting a premium service out in front of your usual service, you are back end fronting—taking a back end product or service and putting it in front of your main service to attract a different clientele into your sphere of influence.

Now you begin to better understand my missed opportunities when I was in practice. I had all these cool techniques and approaches I could have marketed to a variety of different audiences, rather than my standard "here's how chiropractic works and what's in it for you" kind of talk.

Active Release Technique (ART)

Another extremity technique deserving of mention as a back end front is ART, Active Release Technique (activerelease.com), developed by Dr. Michael Leahy. Many chiropractors use it as a primary technique, but you can use it for back-end fronting if you do promotions about those conditions, and bring in new patients who can then be exposed to the array of services and products you provide, again, in the context of their own needs and wants.

Contact Reflex Analysis (CRA)

I didn't know Dr. Dick Versendaal when I was in practice other than to admire him from afar, but I got to know him when he was advising my partners on some serious health problems, and their responses were miraculous and awe-inspiring. Dr. V., founder of Contact Reflex Analysis (CRAwellness.com), turned out to be a brilliant resource of technique, philosophy, and practical clinical knowledge.

He developed his own line of natural oils and herbal supplements, Vervita (vervita.com), and between the potency and showmanship of his flashy technique and the profit centers from the products, CRA offers a natural back-end fronting opportunity. You can do talks, mall shows, engage other professionals in network or write blogs, articles and newsletters about your amazing results. It's a direct route to convert new patients who are attracted to CRA to the other services and products you offer. Dr. V is no longer with us, but his work lives on as a significant legacy that is still unfolding.

Natural Force Healing

I have known and admired Dr. Ken Davis (davisahs.com) since he was my technique instructor at New York Chiropractic College in 1977. He is a master of AK, SOT, nutrition, Rees's soft tissue orthopedics, harmonics, and a cornucopia of discoveries he and his wife Lisa have evolved.

The sum total of his thirty-five years of research is Natural Force Healing, which makes a good back end front for a traditional chiropractor because it encapsulates elements of many advanced technique procedures into a consistent system. It can be promoted through lecture, e-publications, and screenings.

Koren Specific Technique (KST)

Dr. Tedd Koren (teddkorenseminars.com) is renowned for his vast knowledge of chiropractic philosophy, science, and patient education, but of late he has taken the technique world by storm with his magical Koren Specific Technique. Having suffered some serious health issues no one could seem to help him with, he developed KST by combining Van Rumpt's Directional Non Force Technique (DNFT), which happened to be my own primary technique, and Lowell Ward's spinal stressology, which I believe had its roots in the Truscott Angular Adjusting System, as described by Granville Frisbie—obscure techniques and references, perhaps, but seminal influences on chiropractic technique from the crevices of history, dug out, dusted off, rejuvenated, and synthesized by Tedd to create a technique sensation

KST is a non-forceful technique that is performed with an adjusting instrument while the patient is standing, so it is a perfect addition to any chiropractor's technique arsenal.

All of these advanced techniques—CRT, Mally Extremity Technique, Functional Neurology, ART, CRA, Natural Force Healing, NRC, and KST—are powerful techniques that many doctors use as their primary techniques. But the opportunity exists to use any or all of these as options in addition to your mainstream chiropractic approach.

By positioning these techniques as specialties, you can add another layer of services that attract a different clientele, either to enjoy that specialty, or to stick around to appreciate more of your services, including regular chiropractic care.

Foot Levelers

A common back end item in many offices is the foot orthosis, known colloquially as orthotics. My favorite brand is Foot Levelers, since their objective is to set the foot in motion rather than to fix it in place. I also strongly support Kent Greenawalt, whom I perceive to be one of the most important people in chiropractic, both because of his own philanthropy and his leadership through the Foundation for Chiropractic Progress.

I recommend scanning every patient on the way in as part of your entry exam, whether you fit the patient for orthotics at that time or not. By baselining the foot structure, you have a way to observe any changes, and if you believe that foot support is essential for optimal spinal health and therefore brain and nerve system health, then building a system around offering your patients Foot Levelers makes sense.

To put the back end up front, you can place a display in your reception area, do a talk on the value of orthotics, or even take a booth at a health fair—people often see the relevance and value of this kind of product, and it is easy to segue the conversation from foot structure to spinal structure to brain and nerve system function.

Serum Thiol Testing

One of my first chiropractic heroes was Guy Riekeman, whom I first met as a chiropractic student in 1976, sitting in Gary Dalto and Eileen Rose's backyard where I first heard about the predicament of the species, the drama of the mystery of life, and the other foundational Renaissance principles.

Dr. Riekeman is one of our great chiropractic communicators, and during his Renaissance days, he spoke of an eco-geneticist named Ron Pero, who was researching the chemistry of genetic expression. He had made some great discoveries about the effect of chiropractic care that were never clearly defined except to say they were positive.

It wasn't until over thirty years later that I heard of David Walls-Kaufman and Clay Campbell, who apparently had continued with Pero's research and now were prepared to bring it to the chiropractic marketplace.

Here's the amazing breakthrough in a nutshell.

It seems that Pero realized there was a substance in the blood called thiol that was part of the DNA repair mechanism, so it was intimately involved in the healing and aging process. He could predict the probability of serious disease by the level of serum thiol he could measure.

His research demonstrated that having too little thiol forecast a 95% chance of suffering serious illnesses, like cancer or heart disease, and that having sufficient thiol dropped that probability to 5%, a nineteen-fold decrease.

The early scientists analyzed many blood samples, and virtually all of them were thiol deficient, so they had to project and speculate about the trajectory of human health—they had no examples of people with enough thiol, though they saw the possibility of it.

It wasn't until a chance meeting with Joe Flesia, Guy Riekeman's partner in Renaissance, that Pero was posed with the possibility that there was something that seemed to consistently raise thiol levels—chiropractic care.

This is the holy grail of chiropractic research—not that back pain and blood pressure studies aren't productive and validating, because they surely are.

But proving that chiropractic care slows the aging process by facilitating DNA replication and repair, well, that's a whole new level. It means that chiropractic is truly a natural way to health, based not only on chiropractic philosophy, but on science as well. That makes serum thiol testing an incredible back end front. If you want to include serum thiol testing as a predictor of a patient's tendency toward serious illness and track their movement toward wellness, contact The Masters Circle.

Food Allergy Testing

Food allergy is one of the most prevalent issues in health, yet for most people, their status is unclear—if they don't have an obvious negative response to a foodstuff, they think they're okay, but this is often not the case.

Dr. Brian Wolfs in Toronto (hemocode.com) has developed a program where you can test for 250 food intolerances, providing a significant window into your patient's metabolism and offering a profound opportunity to refine their food intake and help them avoid stepping on any biochemical land mines. And since food allergies are so prevalent, it sets up a natural back end front, through talks, mailings, an e-blast, or whatever.

Coupons and Certificates

A quick word about coupons and certificates. Many doctors are creating a lot of new traffic through their offices with coupon promotions like Groupon and Living Social. When a chiropractor offers a massage promotion, or a personal training session, or a nutritional consultation, those are all back-end fronting.

If you can develop your own list, you can launch your own coupon promotions—just check your relevant regulations to be sure you don't step over any legal or ethical boundaries.

Integrating Five-by-Five Marketing

In Chapter 5, we talked about Five-by-Five Marketing, which I learned about from Jack Canfield. You can choose five different back-end fronting options, come up with five different methods of promoting each, and use the five-by-five approach to attract new patients every day through back-end fronting. Just pick one, two, or however many action steps you are willing to commit to each day, and see how quickly you attract new patients every day.

Massage	Blog/ newsletter	coupon	mall show	direct mail	referral
Extremities	Blog/ newsletter	talk	YouTube	direct mail	referral
MindFit	Blog/ newsletter	talk	mall show	direct mail	referral
Foot Levelers	Blog/ newsletter	coupon	mall show	direct mail	referral
Serum Thiol	Blog/ newsletter	talk	mall show	YouTube	referral

By expanding on your ideal patient definitions, you can use these back-end fronting techniques to attract those who fit those new descriptions. This will feed into the development of your new patient machine as you make distinctions about what works best, what works okay, and what doesn't work at all for you.

My Second Outcome

You may remember that I began this chapter by talking about two common denominators I noticed in the most successful chiropractors; absolute certainty and emotional engagement. As I mentioned, for my purposes I morphed these qualities into my own format—firstly, to have certainty that on one could walk into my office with a subluxation complex I couldn't figure out.

The second outcome I aimed for was for that patient's visit with me to be the high point of their day. I don't know about you, but my patients tended to be under a lot of stress, and I knew it was up to me to reduce that stress as thoroughly as I could.

I always loved my patients, and treated them like gold. I made sure they knew how much I appreciated the privilege of being their chiropractor. I wanted to be sure they felt appreciated, because I was genuinely grateful for the opportunity to serve them, and that feeling came out in everything I did.

As a result, I constantly got feedback from patients that coming to see me was the high point of their day, my second outcome.

The more we understand and support our patients' values, the more likely they will be happy with our services. We do so many things to help people get well and stay well—let's broaden our influence by reaching out in as many directions as we can to engage people in the chiropractic lifestyle, ultimately including all pertinent aspects of health and wellness care.

Give people the latitude to embrace some element of your service. You clearly think it's valuable, or else you wouldn't offer it in the first place. Let the relationship mature and blossom, develop trust, and advise the patient like you would a close friend or family member. They will sense your authenticity and concern, and your communication will go to a new level.

Through back-end fronting, you can reach deeper into your community and bring more people into the natural way to health. There are many roads to wellness—show people the way in a language they already comprehend, and earn the right to guide them to all the other helpful and valuable methods you believe will serve them well.

Points to Remember

1. Commit to being an expert on finding and correcting subluxation, and make your visit the high point of your patient's day.

2. Your back end, the services and products you offer beyond your basic chiropractic care, are not only a source of additional profit, they can also be put up front to attract patients who might not otherwise be attracted.

Actions to Take

1. Choose a back-end item you think would appeal to people in your community and develop a way to push it up front and promote it primarily.

2. Visit other doctors in your community who have become known for unique aspects of their practices—notice how you could apply similar reasoning and strategy to build your own clientele.

Questions to Ponder

1. Does it offend you to "sell" additional products and services above and beyond your chiropractic care? Why or why not?

2. What would happen in your practice if you made all the different benefits you offer in your practice available to more people who might not otherwise know about them? Do you see how promoting your back end is a thorough way to practice?

This concludes Chapter 7, Back-End Fronting. In the eighth and final chapter, we'll be putting all the pieces together so you can build a New Patient Machine.

CHAPTER 8
Building A New Patient Machine

My first few years in practice, I was very enthusiastic. I had the flame of life in my hands, and I was determined to spread the word and guide people toward living subluxation-free, as many as I could reach.

The problem was, those people tended to fall into two categories; those who caught my message and embraced it, some going on to chiropractic college themselves—and those who engaged marginally or not at all, only to disappear after a few visits, never to be heard from again.

As I matured, my case management improved, my patient education came together, and my craving for new patients gave way to a desire for a more committed, more engaged clientele.

I was prepared to make an investment in those who would meet me half-way, and that meant that I needed fewer new patients to fill my schedule when the typical patient stayed longer.

I realize that this is a personal choice, and that many chiropractors love the thrill of acute care. They choose to reach as many new patients as possible, leaving it to the patient and other health advisors to create more wellness. This of course is fine, if and when it happens by choice and not default.

That's why it's so important to build a new patient machine based on your values, principles, and experiences caring for a variety of people. As you make distinctions about which patients you choose to serve at this time, you will adjust your new patient machine to turn out patients who meet those contemporaneous needs.

Let's recap what we've covered in the previous seven chapters so we are prepared to build your new patient machine.

In Chapter 1, we explored the dynamics of new patient acquisition. We realized that to bring in new patients every day, you must have sufficient capacity to receive new patients every day, and then you must generate the attraction to fill that capacity.

In Chapter 2, we role-played the referral scenario, and provided many examples of effective referral technique. In Chapter 3, we refined and expanded the referral process to develop a professional referral network.

In Chapter 4, we saw how to use public speaking to fill your office with ideal patients, and in Chapter 5, we catalogued the many types of promotions, and designed a system called Five-by-Five Marketing that organizes your daily activities around attracting new patients every day.

Chapter 6 was dedicated to Internet marketing, so you can blend your hunting and farming effectively by using online tools, while Chapter 7 focused on back-end fronting, displaying each aspect of your care in its own light so people can see what you do beyond your standard care, and discover ways for you to serve them that often lead to full engagement.

Now that we've accumulated all these distinctions and techniques, it's time to assemble these moving parts into a new patient machine that will generate new patients every day.

The New Patient Machine

The New Patient Machine requires the interaction of four gears—targeting ideal patients, building new patient capacity, setting effective new patient goals, and developing a marketing calendar that self-corrects and brings in new patients every day.

Let's begin our study of the New Patient Machine by learning how to target your ideal patient.

How To Target Your Ideal Patient

Some doctors are interested in attracting very specific types of patients, such as personal injury patients, children, seniors, or athletes, while some practices are more general in nature, appealing to families, industry, patients with a variety of conditions, or wellness patients who want to be as healthy as possible.

No matter which kinds of patients you like best, one thing is clear ... if you build your practice with patients you enjoy taking care of, you'll have more fun, be more productive, suffer less stress, and be able to handle more volume. Your areas of expertise will be best utilized, and the patients you don't relate to or don't enjoy taking care of will not be attracted to you as often.

Regardless of your preference, there are specific strategies by which you can shape your practice to have the types of patients you like best, and it starts when you begin to identify the types of patients you like.

Step One: Identify Your ideal Patient(s)

Begin to focus on the types of patients you like best. Notice the characteristics of those you find more desirable. For example, age or gender may play a role ... do you prefer to take care of men, or women? If so, write it down. Do you like to take care of kids, or seniors, or people about your own age? Think for a moment, then write down your impressions.

You're beginning to create a model of an ideal patient that will help you decide how to market yourself in your community. The reason we're concentrating on developing this model is because if you love taking care of kids, you won't find them in a seniors' home ... you have to go to schools, PTAs, and parenting groups, or network with pediatricians and obstetricians.

If you like helping athletes with sports injuries, you have to look in health clubs, not in attorneys' offices. By having a clearly defined model of the kinds of patients you want, your marketing strategy becomes clearer.

Now, consider your overall practice philosophy. Do you prefer the thrill of acute or emergency care, and the satisfaction of bailing patients out who really got themselves in trouble? Or, do you prefer longer-term wellness patients who come to see you on a regular basis to get healthy and stay healthy throughout their lives? It should be obvious enough that both approaches are essential in any community, but do you, in particular, like one type better? If you'd like a blend, what proportion would you like?

Write down your distinctions ... acute and emergency care or longer-term wellness patients. Next, consider the patients' socio-economics. Do you enjoy helping white-collar businesspeople, or would you rather take care of blue-collar working people? Do you relate better to middle-class families, or to a more affluent clientele? Are you compelled to serve the underprivileged, or would you prefer to rub shoulders with your community's elite?

240

Once again, none of these are right or wrong. The purpose of this exercise is not to judge people, or yourself for that matter, but rather to decide on your favorite types of patients so you can look forward to going to your office every single day and taking care of the patients you enjoy most.

Write down the socio-economic group or groups you prefer ... lower, lower-middle, middle, upper-middle or upper class. Recognize that you'll have to market differently to middle-class families than you will to upper-middle-class businesspeople ... that's the reason you're specifying the groups you like best.

There may be certain types of conditions you really like to deal with, or problems you get great results with—or, you may prefer a patient who isn't there for any kind of painful disorder, but who wants chiropractic as health and wellness care. Begin to specify your preferences.

Do you feel confident when a headache patient walks into your office? Or, do you have specialized training in disc cases, or chronic degenerative problems? Do you love when a carpal tunnel patient comes to your office looking to avoid surgery? Have you studied advanced techniques that give you tools to help people with organic problems? If you really like taking care of patients with certain conditions, write them down, and if you'd really rather that people came to you for wellness care regardless of their present condition, write that down, too. You are formulating your model of the ideal patient according to you so you can market yourself appropriately and create a practice that you build based on your desires.

How about financial responsibility? Some doctors prefer that patients pay directly on a per-visit or per-year basis, the cash practice approach. Some doctors would prefer to use an assignment system, working with insurance carriers and having patients responsible only for deductibles and co-payments. Still others choose to work with workers' compensation or personal injury patients so that attorneys and third-party payers handle the financial management of cases. Each style has its advantages and pit-falls, but you probably have a preference. Decide if your ideal patient is a cash patient, an insurance assignment patient, a workers' compensation patient, a personal injury patient, or a Medicare patient, or some combination of those, and write it down.

You may also want to consider the specific physical characteristics of patients. Some doctors find it difficult to take care of very large patients, while some doctors enjoy them. Some doctors prefer muscular, athletic patients, while others find it a challenge to examine and adjust people with thick musculature. Some doctors have very firm techniques, and would rather have a sturdy patient than a fragile older person or a young child. Decide if there are any specifically desirable or undesirable physical characteristics of patients, and write them down.

Sometimes, doctors really enjoy taking care of patients in a particular occupation or industry, or like patients who share a common interest or hobby. Do you relate to people who work with their hands, or highly educated people who can carry a philosophical discussion? Do you love taking care of golfers or tennis players? Do you like body builders, or bowlers, or people who like to cook or read poetry?

Attracting people who have common interests creates another area of rapport that makes you feel more connected to your patients. Also, you may have specific insights into their situation that may help you to take better care of them than someone without your experience or expertise.

Do you love stressed-out, hyper businesspeople because they want the fastest adjustment possible and never waste thirty seconds of your time? Or do you like aerobics instructors who love to discuss the finer points of exercise physiology? Do you enjoy industrial relations, and doing hazard and risk analyses at factories, or taking care of repetitive motion disorder or low back lifting accidents? Decide if there are any occupations, hobbies, or interests that would make a patient more desirable for your practice, and write them down now.

Does your technique lend itself to certain types of clientele? Do you use a light force approach that appeals to aficionados, or caters to cowards, seniors, or kids? Do you really like to feel the bones move under your hands? Are you interested in using nutrition, exercise, cranial work, organ techniques, or energy balancing? Or do you prefer the pure and simple approach? There are as many techniques as there are chiropractors, and some patients will respond better to your approach than others. Decide what types of patients would be most responsive to your technique, and write them down.

At this point, you may be starting to notice some patterns here. Clearly, there are going to be some patients who are very well suited to your practice and you to them—and, there are going to be some patients who are just not ideal for you, and vice versa. Remember, this is not about judging people as better or worse, but rather to focus on attracting the people you prefer, for those times when you have a choice.

Some of you may be thinking, "Can't I just serve whoever comes in?" The answer is—of course! No practice consists entirely of ideal patients, and indeed, you may learn valuable lessons from patients who are outside your optimal patient definition.

This exercise is designed to help you decide how to spend your marketing time, energy, and money to increase the percentage of ideal patients and ideal referrals. You may think of yourself as a generalist who takes all comers, and that is fine, if you're flexible enough to enjoy all kinds of people.

Most doctors, though, find certain kinds of patients gratifying, and others draining. This process helps you identify those patients you like best, when you do have a preference. After all, if you can see a certain number of people each day, why not make as many of them ideal patients as possible?

Now you have a list of characteristics of your favorite kinds of patients. Think about what you have discovered about your choices, and continue working on these ideal patient models to get crystal-clear about what you like best. You may find that you have two or three kinds of patients that meet your criteria in their own way, and that's fine.

Get a clear picture of your ideal patients, and the ones you don't like as much. The ones you don't like may be better off somewhere else anyway, so you can make room for the ones you like best. There's no shortage of potential patients—they're everywhere you look! That's why it makes sense to decide which kinds you like best, and shape your marketing around them.

You can use these distinctions as a checklist for your basic model:

- personal characteristics, like age, gender, or size
- socio-economics
- types of conditions
- practice philosophy on acute or wellness care
- method of payment
- occupations, hobbies, or common interests
- patients who require or respond to specialized techniques

You may come up with other aspects of ideal patients that are important to you. Add them to your descriptions to enrich the detail, and focus your mind on what you really want. As a matter of fact, this exercise may remind you of patients already in your practice who fit some or all of these criteria. Pick out about five of your favorite patients.

Which categories do they fall into? Are there other criteria you really prefer that aren't yet on your lists? Make your descriptions as detailed as possible, because they will help you identify and attract the right patients for you.

Step Two: Locate Your Ideal Patients

Now that you know which kinds of patients you are looking for, you have to determine where this type of patient is most likely to be found. Think about your ideal patient—is he or she a young, athletic health freak with two little children and a passion for tennis? This person is likely to be found in a tennis or health club, a health food store or parenting group. Do you prefer seniors with chronic problems? This individual can be found through seniors' homes, adult services, and home care groups, or through referrals from other professionals who serve this population.

Can you see the futility of marketing seniors' homes if what you really like is young athletes? Now you understand why that can't work. So, once you've decided who you want, think about where they are.

Where is your ideal patient most likely to work? Write down possible places of employment. Where does he or she tend to meet socially? Write down any gathering places that may apply. Which civic organizations could he or she belong to? Write them down, too. What hobbies might he or she pursue? Write down the establishments that your ideal patient may frequent. At what religious or ethnic meeting places might he or she be? Are there particular neighborhoods where there are many potential ideal patients for you?

You want to fish in a fishing hole that has the kind of fish you're fishing for. Brainstorm all the possible places where your ideal patients may be and write them down so you can proceed to the next step, and that is to increase your visibility at these targeted areas.

Step Three: Increase Your Visibility

There are many ways to increase your visibility so your ideal patients can find you. If possible, and appropriate, you may want to join and participate yourself. For example, if you love sports and enjoy working with athletes, then join the local club or gym and increase your presence there. Or, if there's a particular religious or ethnic group that you relate to, attend their meetings and participate that way. As you become personally involved, the people there become more comfortable and familiar with you, and it's more likely that they'll choose someone they know and like.

Or, you may want to arrange for some speaking engagements. Doing a presentation serves the dual purpose of providing information and also establishing you as an authority on your chosen topic of discussion. If you like industrial relations and workers' compensation patients, a group presentation is an excellent way to increase your visibility. If your target location is a health club, you may want to do a series of talks, including topics like the role of the brain, spine, and nerve system in exercise, nutrition, safe workouts, stress reduction, health philosophy, or even classes on preventing or dealing with different types of athletic injury.

Or, you can go to a seniors' home and do presentations on aging gracefully, life extension, arthritis, osteoporosis, or other related health issues, such as dealing with Medicare, coping with an ailing spouse, or fighting age prejudice. The idea is not only to teach, but also to meet the needs of the population you want to work with, to let them know you're focused on them, and that you care.

Another technique is to use their communications network to advertise your message. For example, if there's any in-house newsletter or bulletin, see if you can write a column on interesting health-related issues. Or, advertise in the bulletin, if they accept ads, or sponsor a particular edition in conjunction with a holiday or special event of some sort.

Some doctors have found businesses receptive to distributing fliers in employees' pay envelopes. Occasionally, they'll even do a mailing to promote your presentations or introduce you to the staff. However you can swing it, try to get the administration of your targeted location to endorse you in some very obvious way.

Another good idea is to refer your patients to these places. Firstly, you help your patient by making a connection that will benefit him or her. Secondly, you now have an agent on the inside, talking you up and spreading the good word. So, if you want more kids in your practice, then think, where are the kids? They're at school, at camp, on sports teams, or at the pediatrician's office.

To market for kids, you can do presentations at school, refer a couple of your teenage patients to be counselors at camp, provide the coach with some handouts on preventing or proper care of common injuries to distribute to the team members, or refer young families to the pediatrician for checkups or medical services if necessary, so the pediatrician gets to hear how terrific you are from someone who's not you. Are you starting to get the idea?

You can also increase your visibility with specific targeted advertising, and this can be done in several ways. If there is a publication that targets a group you like, for example an ethnic newspaper, or a newsletter from a local service organization you relate to, you can run advertisements or articles that position you as an authority.

Or, you can buy mailing lists that demographically target your ideal patients in your community and send specific materials directly to their homes. Or, you can do some advertising in a regional newspaper, and focus the ad on attracting a certain type of patient. Or, you can take the lists you bought and do some telemarketing.

Or, use your creativity to come up with novel and exciting ways to provide value for your target group. Remember, the idea here is to increase your visibility, so anything you can do that puts you in a positive light with your potential ideal patients is probably the right thing to do.

Now that you've identified your ideal patient, located your ideal patient, and increased your visibility in those target areas, it's time to talk about closing.

Step Four: Close Effectively

Closing means getting the person to say, "Yes, I would like to be your patient," and without this step, all the rest of this is nothing more than exercise. The point here is to fill up your office with great patients, so learning to close properly is an essential part of the process.

You have to have an appropriate closing prepared for any eventuality. Here is a good strategy for planning your closing. First, imagine the setting for the closing—a closing to a group after a presentation will be different from a one-on-one with an employer or a health club manager, and those will be different still from closing a neighborhood attorney or pediatrician. You have to custom-tailor your closing to the situation, so play the situation in your imagination and write out (or at least plan out) your complete script for the projected scenario so you can refine and master it.

Once you have your basic script prepared, then you need to rehearse it so when you do it in a real-life situation, it comes out smooth and professional. Make your mistakes in rehearsal, so when it's time to close the ideal patient for real, you've got it down.

Here is a simple and effective strategy for closing. First, summarize the main points of your presentation. Then, show the person or group the benefits of being your patient, and the consequences of not being your patient. Finally, provide an opportunity for the person to say yes by asking a properly formed closing question.

If you are addressing an aerobics class, for example, your closing might sound something like this:

"So, what did we talk about here today? Well, we talked about health, and what it takes to be healthy. We talked about the important role exercise and proper nutrition play in your health. We also talked about your brain, nerve system, and spine, and how your spinal function can affect all aspects of your well-being. Finally, we talked about how keeping your nerve system healthy can improve your health and your quality of life.

"Now some of you may be thinking, 'You mean if I get chiropractic care, then my spine will be more flexible, my muscles will have a strong and balanced framework to grow on, I'll feel better and my body will work better?' While others may be thinking, 'You mean that spinal distortion isn't only unpleasant to look at, but can cause pain and prevent normal body function and normal workouts, eventually decreasing mobility until the degenerative process fuses the misaligned vertebrae, never to move properly again?'

"Whatever you're thinking, you've probably realized that chiropractic care can help you! For those of you who would like to be examined to find out specifically what's going on in your body, my assistant Mary has an appointment book at the back of the room, so please make your appointment before you leave ... and, for those of you who have a question, please come up as we break and I'll be glad to answer it so you'll know everything you need to know about getting chiropractic care for you and your family. Thank you very much for your attention, and please make your appointments before you go."

Now, did you catch the four parts to the closing? Go back over the script and mark out the four parts, and practice inserting other language, benefits, consequences, and choices in the closing so you become skillful at fitting this closing into any scenario.

When you target a certain type of patient, use illustrations and metaphors that match that particular group. Notice that for an aerobics class you can talk about appearance, flexibility, and balance. For young families, talk about having fun together, saving money on health costs by avoiding problems due to brain, spine, and nerve system neglect, and growing up strong and healthy. For an employer, you could talk about increasing employee productivity and decreasing workplace stress. You might also discuss getting injured workers back on the job with less expense and inconvenience.

No matter what, make your closing more powerful by evoking an emotional response from the particular audience you are addressing.

Step Five: Custom-Tailor Your Office Procedure

Finally, now that you've targeted, located, engaged, and closed your ideal patient, remember to organize your office procedure to suit these types of patients. For example, don't sit a stressed-out executive in front of a half-hour video, and don't schedule a five-minute consultation/history/ examination for a senior. If you like young families, have something in the reception area for the kids to do, and so on.

You see, the sky's the limit when you target your ideal patient. By focusing on the kinds of patients you like best, you'll create a practice you enjoy going to every day. With as many ideal patients as possible, you'll build a practice that is truly ideal for you.

Here's a worksheet to help you organize your efforts.

HOW TO TARGET YOUR IDEAL PATIENT SUMMARY

To fill your office with the kind of patients you most want to take care of:

1. Specifically describe, in writing, the exact kind of patient(s) you prefer:

    a. acute care/regular care

    b. philosophical orientation

    c. types of conditions

    d. socio-economics

    e. age/gender

    f. employment

    g. specific characteristics (desirable/undesirable)

    h. PI/WC/Insurance/$

2. Determine where this kind of patient is most likely to be found:

    a. places of employment

    b. social gathering places

    c. civic organizations

    d. hobbies

    e. religious/ethnic meeting places

    f. particular neighborhoods

    g. specific locations

3. Increase your visibility at those targeted areas in the form of:

    a. joining them yourself

    b. arranging speaking engagements

    c. using their house organ or newsletter

    d. specific targeted advertising

e. referring people already under your care to these places, both for their benefit and also to represent you

f. specific targeted telemarketing

g. use your creativity to generate value for the group

h. Internet marketing

4. Have an appropriate closing prepared for any eventuality:

a. write a complete script for the projected scenario

b. rehearse the most usual scenes for smoothness and professionalism

c. four-part closing technique—summarize, toward, away, bind

d. manage the process by using the "How to do anything" format

   • state—get into a resourceful state

   • outcome—know your desired outcome

   • sensory acuity—notice if your actions move you toward or away from outcome

   • flexibility—vary your actions to move toward your outcome

5. Have a well-organized office intake procedure.

The Right New Patient Flow For You

Now that you know how to target your ideal patient, we need to analyze your new patient capacity with an exercise called "The Right New Patient Flow For You."

Everyone has a different optimal new patient flow. Remember that new patient flow is an effect, not a cause, and most usually, a chiropractor would do better to work on expanding the capacity of his or her practice than to try to artificially induce a temporary increase in new patient volume.

The purpose of this section, then, is to help you figure out what the right new patient flow is for you at your present capacity, and how to prepare your time management and goal-setting systems to accommodate your growth to your desired capacity.

How do you know how many new patients you need to build your practice to the level you want? I know doctors who have practices of every imaginable volume—practices that see 200 visits a week, practices that see 200 visits a month, practices that see 200 visits on a slow morning—and these practices require different new patient volume to function at those levels.

You see, depending on the way you want to run your practice, there is an ideal number of new patients for you—a number that satisfies you, and grows the practice at the rate you choose, or a number that challenges you, or gives you a feeling of making a difference—and you are the only one who knows what you want to accomplish with your practice.

Think about what size practice you ultimately want, and let's ask a few questions to get us started with the process.

How Many People Do You Want To See Each Day?

How many people do you want to see each day? Twenty? Thirty? Fifty? A hundred? Two hundred?

There's no right or wrong number here—just decide how many you believe you can see right now on a comfortably busy day. As you grow, you'll be able to change these numbers, so just focus on understanding the concepts and learning the systems. Let's use an example of fifty visits a day. Fifty people each day times three full office days and two half-days each week, that would be two hundred office visits each week, or about eight hundred each month.

What is your method of measuring patient compliance and retention? Do this simple math—divide the average number of office visits each month by the average number of new patients each month.

This gives you a measurement known as a Patient Visit Average, or PVA. Once you know your present PVA, you can use this number to predict how many new patients you'd need to get to your target level—just divide your target volume by your PVA to get the number of new patients required.

For example, if you have a 40 PVA, in other words, an average patient stays in your office forty visits, then to get to eight hundred visits, you would need twenty new patients (800 OVs / 40 PVA = 20 NPs.)

If an average patient stays in your office for 25 visits, you would need 32 new patients to get to the same 800 office visits, while if an average patient stays in your office 50 visits, you'd need only 16 to get to 800. (There is no right or wrong PVA—it just reflects your style of practice. A PVA is only inappropriate if it is not consistent with your desired patient compliance.)

I know doctors with PVAs of over 100, who start 4 new patients per week and see 400 office visits, and doctors with a 40 PVA who start 10 new patients per week and see the same 400 office visits. In order for you to begin to figure out the right new patient flow for you, decide how many people you want to see, divide by your patient visit average, and that will give you the number of new patients you need to see.

Now, think about how long it would take you to process a new patient if you were really being time efficient.

Add a minute or two just to be on the safe side, and use this time as a reference. Remember that the new patient usually requires two long visits at the beginning of care, the first for consultation and examination, and the second for report of findings and first adjustment. How many of these longer "special" slots can you fit in each day to process new people, and still have the time you need to see your regular office visits?

Here's where you start to plan your ideal office day.

If you want to see fifty people, for example, and you work from 9-12 and 2-6, that's seven office hours each day. If you can see ten office visits per hour, then that would take five hours, leaving you two hours to process new people and handle your other administrative work. So, if at a 40 PVA you need 5 new patients per week to be at 50 visits a day, then you have to plan 10 special slots per week, or 2 to 3 each day.

Are you starting to see why it's so important to look at this? If you only have time to schedule one special slot each day, then you won't have the capacity in your schedule to start the number of new patients you need to get to the volume you want. By understanding this, you can begin to use your time more efficiently, and thereby expand your capacity.

Your Capacity Determines Your Volume

As we discussed in Chapter 1, the mechanics of your office must support the new patient flow you want, and you must be able to conceptualize or envision the desired new patient flow. You must believe that it's possible to see the number of new patients you'd need to get to your target volume, and you must be, or be willing to become, the kind of person who can handle that new patient flow. This combination of your ability to perform and your beliefs about your performance will determine your capacity.

I remember having a spirited debate with a dear friend and colleague early in both of our careers. "You can't see 100 people a day and give quality care," he fumed—and then, a year or so later, when he was doing it, I reminded him of our conversation. "Oh," he said, "that was who I was then—I'm different now." And how right he was—for in those few words, he summed up the capacity challenge—your capacity will be limited or expanded by who you believe yourself to be; in other words, by your identity.

Consider this—if I come to your office and take over for you, without changing anything else, keeping the same location, same staff, same equipment, even the same competition in town, you can be sure that within a very short period of time, that practice will be different from when you were running it.

Maybe it'll be busier, maybe slower, but one thing is certain—that practice will reflect the doctor who's in charge, because, Doctor, like it or not, your practice is you. So, if you want to grow your practice, you have to grow yourself, to grow your identity.

The right new patient flow for you is going to be based in part on the number of new patients you believe you can see, and the personal and professional qualities you bring to the new patient process. Let's integrate these ideas to see how to calculate the right new patient flow for you.

Take a look at the Right New Patient Flow Worksheet:

RIGHT NEW PATIENT FLOW WORKSHEET

Baseline Office Parameters

A. Present PVA = average monthly OVs / average monthly NPs = __ PVA

B. Comfortably busy day = _____ OVs

C. # office days per month = _____ days / month

D. Present OV capacity = B x C = _____ OVs / month

E. Present NP capacity = D / A = _____ NPs

Time Capacity Evaluation

F. # OVs / hour = _____ OVs / hour

G. # hours to see present OV capacity = D / F = _____ hours

H. Total office hours per month = _____ hours / month

I. # hours you have for other than OVs = H - G = _____

J. # hours to process NP (first time visits) = _____ hour(s)

K. Present NP Time Capacity I / J = _____ NPs

If K is more than or equal to E, then you can handle this NP flow, based on your present use of time and resources. If not, then look at capacity limitations, such as current PVA, amount of time spent processing OVs and/or NPs, whether or not certain functions can be delegated, which resources may need to be built, etc.

Desired Volume Projection

L. Desired OV volume per month = _____ OVs / month

M. Desired OV volume per day = L / C = _____ OVs / day

N. Desired NP flow = L / A = _____ NPs

O. # hours to see desired OV volume = L / F = _____ hours

P. # hours for other than OVs = H - O = _____ hours

Q. Desired NP time capacity = P / J = _____ NPs

If Q is more than or equal to N, then you can handle this NP flow based on your present use of time and resources. If not, then look at capacity limitations, such as current PVA, amount of time spent processing OVs and/or NPs, whether or not certain functions can be delegated, which resources may need to be built, etc.)

If your practice is you, then your volume will depend on your capacity. Figure out your present capacity this way—take your average number of office visits per month, and divide by your present average number of new patients per month. This is your present patient visit average, or PVA.

Think of what a nice, comfortably busy office day would feel like—about how many office visits would you like to see? Take this number and multiply it by the number of office days in a month—for example, if you work three full and two half-days each week, that would be about 16 days per month.

That gives you your present monthly office visit capacity. Divide that number by your PVA, and that gives you your present new patient capacity.

Check to see that you could schedule all the office visits and special slots you'd need to get to this volume. If not, decide whether it's a limitation in capacity by procedure, such as time management, staff training, or clarity of office policy, or an issue of capacity by concept and vision, such as self-image, fear of confrontation or rejection, poor attitude, or inadequate leadership. By identifying your weaker areas, you'll be able to focus your energy where it's needed to bring yourself up to your present capacity.

Think about how many office visits you'd like to see in a month. That number will represent your desired monthly office visit capacity. Divide that number by your PVA to give you your desired monthly new patient capacity. Divide these numbers by 4 to get the weekly numbers, and by 16 to get the daily numbers.

Do you see why we did all this calculation? We have to make sure that it's possible for you to see that number of office visits per day and start that number of new patients each week—otherwise, you have set goals for yourself that are not appropriate for your present stage of development.

And, if you realize that you can definitely handle that volume, then that belief, that sense of certainty, will make it more likely that you will.

The point is this—we may throw numbers around that are nothing more than wishes and hopes, and get us no closer to our desired volume, because we don't have the capacity to handle that number of people on a daily basis. To avoid being frustrated by unrealistic or inappropriate goals, we have to check to be sure it's possible to schedule all the appointments we need, and also get all of our other work done—and, we also have to believe that it's possible to see that number of people, so our self-concept matches up with the goal structure we want.

That way, you can be sure that the new patient flow you are aiming for will get you to your target volume, and also will not overburden either your daily procedures or your self-concept, so the growth is enjoyable instead of stressful. As you grow, both through refining your procedures and expanding your identity, you'll find that the number of new patients you want will fluctuate, depending on your goals at that particular time. But, by using these methods of evaluation, you'll always have a way of determining the right new patient flow for you.

Here are two examples to illustrate how you can use this analysis to be certain you can handle the number of new patients you desire. In this example, this doctor is currently seeing 16 new patients, and has a time capacity for 32.

RIGHT NEW PATIENT FLOW WORKSHEET: Example 1

Baseline Office Parameters

A. Present PVA = average monthly OVs / average monthly NPs = 40 PVA

B. Comfortably busy day = 40 OVs

C. # office days per month = 16 days / month

D. Present OV capacity = B x C = 640 OVs / month

E. Present NP capacity = D / A = 16 NPs

Time Capacity Evaluation

F. # OVs / hour = 8 OVs / hour

G. # hours to see present OV capacity = D / F = 80 hours

H. Total office hours per month = 112 hours / month

I. # hours you have for other than OVs = H - G = 32 hours

J. # hours to process NP (first two visits) = 1 hour(s)

K. NP time capacity = I / J = 32 NPs

So, there is ample time to see this number of NPs and still have time to handle paperwork, hold staff meetings, and accomplish other office functions. Also, there is some time to grow—let's see how much room, without changing any of the current parameters. Let's look at increasing the volume 20%, to 768 OVs per month.

Desired Volume Projection

L. Desired OV volume per month = 768 OVs / month

M. Desired OV volume per day = L / C = 48 OVs / day

N. Desired NP flow = L / A = 19-20 NPs

O. # hours to see desired OV volume = L / F = 96 hours

P. # hours for other than OVs = H - O = 16 hours

Q. NP time capacity = P / J = 16 NPs)

When Q, the new patient time capacity, is less than N, the desired new patient flow, your capacity is less than your goal, so there isn't sufficient time in the doctor's schedule to handle all of the work that needs to be done. Now you can see why this doctor cannot sustain this increase in volume—some aspect of time capacity is limiting the growth. Where might the weaker areas be?

You can increase the efficiency of your NP processing, improve the use of your appointment book so you can see more patients per hour, streamline your office visit, increase your PVA with the PVA skills, work more hours, or delegate some of the responsibilities to an assistant or associate.

Now let's look at the effect of seeing 10 visits/hour instead of 8.

RIGHT NEW PATIENT FLOW WORKSHEET: Example 2

Baseline Office Parameters

A. Present PVA = average monthly OVs / average monthly NP's = 40 PVA

B. Comfortably busy day = 40 OVs

C. # office days per month = 16 days / month

D. Present OV capacity = B x C = 640 OVs / month

E. Present NP capacity = D / A = 16 NPs

Time Capacity Evaluation

F. # OVs / hour = 10 OVs / hour

G. # hours to see present OV capacity = D / F = 64 hours

H. Total office hours per month = 112 hours / month

I. # hours you have for other than OVs = H - G = 48 hours

J. # hours to process NP (first two visits) = 1 hour(s)

K. NP time capacity = I / J = 48 NPs)

So, there is ample time to see this number of NPs and still have time to handle paperwork, hold staff meetings, and accomplish other office functions. Also, there is some time to grow—let's see how much room, with no specific capacity limitations addressed. Now let's look at increasing the volume 20% to 768 OVs/month.

Desired Volume Projection

L. Desired OV volume per month = 768 OVs / month

M. Desired OV volume per day = L / C = 48 OVs / day

N. Desired NP flow = L / A = 19-20 NPs

O. # hours to see desired OV volume = L / F = 76.8 hours

P. # hours for other than OVs = H - O = 33.2 hours

Q. NP time capacity = P / J = 33.2 NPs

Now, there is plenty of time capacity to handle the increase in NPs, just by increasing the tempo of office visits from 8 per hour to 10 per hour. Notice that growing PVA, decreasing processing time for new patients, and delegating non-essential tasks also have a profound effect on time capacity.

Start thinking about how your practice can be evaluated this way—by aiming at the right new patient flow, you will avoid unnecessary frustration and develop more certainty about your goal structure. While this exercise requires you to be analytical, it will reward your hard work with clarity about where your attention is best invested.

The 10%/20% Rule

The third component of the new patient machine is the 10%/20% rule. First, we had to target our ideal patient, to identify the kind of people we want to attract. Then, we evaluated time capacity, to make sure we have a series of strategies and procedures, as well as the beliefs and attitudes that will work for those kinds of people, at the rate and magnitude that we desire.

Now, we have to learn how to set effective goals in a system that capitalizes on the natural momentum of our growth.

The Natural Momentum of Your Growth

Imagine you're trying to cross a river, and you see that there are stones a few feet apart that form a loose path you could use to get to the other side. You could jump from the shore to the first stone, from the first to the second, from the second to the third and so on, each time starting from a standstill and landing with a thud, only to repeat the process again until you get across.

Or, you could observe the spacing of the stones, and begin walking across the river in a smooth, calculated gait, shortening or lengthening your stride when necessary, but moving steadily and without undue effort or friction until you get to the other side.

Clearly both of these strategies would work, but the first is herky-jerky, inefficient, and exhausting, while the second is fluid and effortless, capitalizing on the natural momentum of your movement.

Running Through First Base

At some point you've probably either played or seen a baseball game, so you know that when the batter puts the ball in play, he or she would run to first base, trying to get there before being tagged out.

In baseball's early days, though, a lot of batters were getting thrown out at first, because in order to land safely on first base, they had to start slowing down about halfway there, and that gave the fielders an advantage.

So, the rules were changed so that a batter can run past first base and not be tagged out, so they could run full speed all the way to first base. Once batters could run *through* first base instead of *to* first base, they were able to make it safely more of the time.

Why Many People Don't Reach Their Goals

Hidden in these two stories are a pair of concepts that will revolutionize your goal setting.

Most people set goals by just picking numbers that seem right. Sometimes this works, but often it's too sloppy to apply the vibrational infrastructure and universal forces that make some goals magically appear. It isn't any more complicated to act consistently with such magic, as long as you know what to look for and how to use it.

There are two factors that go into creating a goal—believability and motivation. For a goal to come into your reality, you must believe you can manifest it, and you must be motivated to do whatever it takes to manifest it.

Notice that if your goal is too far out in the distance, it may be very motivating, but maybe not so believable. And if your goal is too close to where you are, it will be very believable, but not very motivating. The best goals are close enough to be believable, and far away enough to be motivating, so they meet both of these criteria.

My observation, after studying numerous goal-setting systems and working with thousands of clients, is that your start point for evaluating your optimal rate of growth should be about 20%. For some people and at some times, it may be appropriate to stretch and aim higher, and under some circumstances a more modest target should be established. For this discussion, I'm going to start with a goal of 20% growth.

Now think about the base runner, slowing down to land right on first base. If you think of your goal as a static target, then as you approach it you'll subconsciously slow down, to try to land right on it.

Instead of running to your goal, run through it. Instead of slowing down halfway there, speed up! Don't wait to hit your goal to raise it; raise it when you get halfway there, so you zoom through your goal and pick up speed, capitalizing on the natural momentum of your growth.

Now you can arrange your goals sequentially, like stepping stones, so you stride across them gracefully and purposefully, crossing the river to get to your ideal practice volume.

Applying The 10%/20% Rule

The best way to set your goals for your office is to aim for 20% growth, and when you get halfway there, or 10% growth, bump the goal another 20%—hence, the 10%/20% rule. This creates an ongoing progression of goals that act as stepping stones to move in the direction you want to grow.

Waiting until you hit the goal interrupts the natural flow of your momentum, so bump the goal at the "bump point"—halfway to your goal, or 10% growth. This preserves the natural momentum of your growth. Look at this example:

Sample 10%/20% Rule

Present volume 400 OVs/month
Next goal level 400 OVs/month + 20% = 480 OVs/month
Bump point 400 OVs/month + 10% = 440 OVs/month
New goal 440 OVs/month + 20% = 528 OVs/month
New bump point 440 OVs/month + 10% = 484 OVs/month
New goal 484 OVs/month + 20% = 581 OVs/month
New bump point 484 OVs/month + 10% = 532 OVs/month
Believability = OV goal level/PVA = #NPs
Motivation = OV goal level x OVA = $ Services
Time frame = approximate time it should take to get to bump point based on previous reference experiences.

My current volume is 400 and my direction is 800.

	10% Bump Point	20% New Goal Level	Believability NPs @ 40 PVA	Motivation Svcs @ 40 OVA	Time Frame
START POINT	400	480	12	19,200	by 4/30
WHEN I GET TO	440	528	13	21,120	
WHEN I GET TO	484	580	14	23,240	
WHEN I GET TO	532	638	16	25,520	
WHEN I GET TO	581	698	17-18	27,920	
WHEN I GET TO	639	767	19	30,680	
WHEN I GET TO	703	844	21	33,760	
WHEN I GET TO	773	928	23	37,120	
WHEN I GET TO	850	1,020	26	40,800	
WHEN I GET TO					
WHEN I GET TO					

So, in this example, let's say your start point is 400 visits per month. Your "right new patient flow" exercise tells you that you can handle up to about 800 visits, so that becomes your direction. Now you want to construct stepwise increments between where you are and where you want to be, spaced properly to maximize and preserve your momentum of growth.

Your first 20% step is to 480 visits—check to see that it is believable, meaning that at the current PVA, in this example 40, it would take 12 new patients to get to 480 visits—is that believable? If yes, then it passes the believability test, and now test the motivation—at a 40 OVA in this example, would an income of 19,200, as compared to the 16,000 at the volume level of 400, would that be motivating? If yes, it passes the motivation test, thereby making it a good goal. If you don't believe you can get there, work on your capacity limitations as described in Chapter 1. If the level isn't motivating, choose a level that is, and then test it for believability. The trick is to make sure your goals are always both believable and motivating.

Your first bump point is halfway there, or 440, so when you hit 440, or even if the first two weeks of the month you see 110 each week, bump the goal then, don't wait until the end of the month. Remember, you are trying to capture momentum, so if you see you've hit the bump point, raise the goal immediately. This brings your goals alive, not just sitting there on a page, but fully engaging you in the process of achieving them.

As you hit each bump point, raise the goal by 20%, or whatever increment you decided upon, and keep moving up in volume as you accomplish each milestone.

Here is a worksheet for you to design your own 10%/20% rule.

10% / 20% RULE WORKSHEET

My present volume is _____ **and my direction is** _____.

	10%	20%	Believability NPs at ___ PVA	Motivation Svcs @ ___ OVA	Time Frame
START POINT					
WHEN I GET TO					
WHEN I GET TO					
WHEN I GET TO					
WHEN I GET TO					
WHEN I GET TO					
WHEN I GET TO					
WHEN I GET TO					
WHEN I GET TO					
WHEN I GET TO					
WHEN I GET TO					

Copy or print out this worksheet and solve your 10%/20% rule by inserting your current volume and your big target, known as your direction. To figure out your believability, divide your 20% goal by your PVA to find how many new patients you need to get there. Do you believe you can get that many? Well, then, good, you've met the believability test for that goal.

Now let's test motivation by multiplying your 20% goal by your OVA, the amount you make per visit. Is it motivating? Well, then, good, your 20%

goal meets both the believability and the motivation test, so it's a good goal.

What if you don't believe you can handle that number of new patients? Go back to the new patient flow exercise and test to see if you have the time capacity. If not, you'll need to streamline your procedures to be able to handle more people in the same time, or expand your office hours, or add an associate—analyze the capacity limitations by procedure and by concept and vision to increase your capacity, and therefore your believability about how much you can handle.

Continue filling in the chart, increasing by 20% and bumping the goal when you get to 10%, or halfway there. Complete the chart until you hit your direction, check it for believability and motivation, and you're ready for the fourth component of the New Patient Machine, The Marketing Calendar.

The Marketing Calendar

The Marketing Calendar is the place where everything we've discussed to date comes together. Once you have targeted your ideal patient, once you have built the capacity to handle what you attract, once you have established a coherent goal structure, and once you have accumulated a rich stockpile of new patient attraction techniques, it's time to organize your new patient acquisition process in the form of a series of directed efforts intended to attract new patients every day, or at whatever rate you choose.

Let's put it all together with a consistent approach, orchestrating your new patient attraction techniques into a specific plan that guides your attention every day, week, and month toward the outcome of bringing in new patients every day.

The construction of such a marketing calendar is relatively simple. Choose a goal for each month, and design new patient marketing techniques to reach that goal and then some. I recommend that you aim ten or twenty percent higher than your goal, just in case some of your new patient generating activities attract fewer actual new patients than expected.

In other words, if you are aiming at 20 new patients a month, plan new patient attraction methods to get to twenty-two or twenty-four new patients as a reasonable hedge to make sure you hit your target.

For each month, draw a box that will represent your marketing calendar for that month. Write the name of the month in the top of the box, and write the goal in the upper right-hand corner and circle it. Let's say, for example, your goal is 20 new patients.

Now, in the middle of the box, write your proposed new patient generating activities, with the goal for each activity written next to it. For example, if you're going to play the three-a-day game, and you expect to attract six new patients from that, write "3/day game" and write the number "6" next to it, and circle it.

Now, if you are planning on doing four health care classes during the month, one each week, and you expect to attract one new patient from each health care class on average, write "4HCC" under "3/day game" and next to it write the number "4" and circle it.

Add more new patient generating activities until you get to at least 22 or 24, to have more certainty that you will get to 20. Make sure you have enough new patient generating activities planned to at least get to your goal.

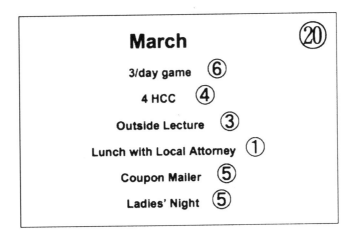

March ⑳

3/day game ⑥

4 HCC ④

Outside Lecture ③

Lunch with Local Attorney ①

Coupon Mailer ⑤

Ladies' Night ⑤

Do this at least several months in advance to allow time to plan and execute those events that are more complex or time-consuming.

Keep track of your goals and results on your monthly marketing calendars. Sequential analysis of your monthly achievements will increase predictability by demonstrating which new patient generating activities are most and least productive so you can direct your time, energy, and capital toward the more productive.

Collect your data from six months of calendars, analyze the degree of productivity of each activity, and reset the next quarter's goals accordingly. Adjust calendars to favor more productive activities so that over time, your marketing process will become more dollar and time productive.

As you continually refine and master this process, you will learn to expect certain results from certain new patient generating activities, and you'll become skillful at interpreting your yield and making smart decisions about where your time, energy, and resources are best invested. Ultimately, this becomes a new patient machine—you turn it on, and it churns out new patients based on your predictions and intentions.

Select goals for each month, and choose specific ways to assign your marketing energy to an assortment of new patient generating activities, chosen from the many tools and techniques presented in this book. Plan enough each month to achieve your goals and then some. Think yearly, quarterly, monthly, weekly, and daily with your NP strategies.

Here's an example of a yearly calendar, showing growth and expansion of new patient generating activities. Notice that this should be done in pencil so you can constantly update and correct it based on your observations, looking backward over the results you've previously achieved. Also, the goals for the first six months are chosen, but the observations made along the way will alter the goals and new patient generating activities, so the calendar can be tweaked in response to that data.

Sample Annual Marketing Calendar

January (20)	February (20)	March (22)
Ask for referrals (12)	Ask for referrals (12)	Ask for referrals (12)
4 HCC (6)	4 HCC (6)	4 HCC (6)
New Year's Resolution Drive (4)	Valentine Promotion (4)	4 Luncheons (3)
		Talk at business (3)

April (22)	May (24)	June (24)
Ask for referrals (10)	Ask for referrals (10)	Ask for referrals (12)
4 HCC (6)	4 HCC (6)	4 HCC (6)
Patient Appreciation Day (8)	Mother's Day Event (10)	Father's Day Event (10)

July	August	September
Ask for referrals	Ask for referrals	Ask for referrals
4 HCC	4 HCC	4 HCC
Health Freedom Day	Back to School Screening	Lecture at PTA
Health Fair	Coupon Mailer	Online Essay Contest

October	November	December
Ask for referrals	Ask for referrals	Ask for referrals
4 HCC	4 HCC	4 HCC
Patient Appreciation Dinner	Thanksgiving Food Drive	Christmas Toy Drive
	Ladies Night of Indulgence	Movie Night

Note that goals for individual projects and promotions only go through half the year to accommodate new distinctions gathered in preparation for the second half. Based on the results, jiggle the goals and expectations to suit the 10%/20% rule.

Don't Forget the Five-by-Five

You can also build your Five-by-Five grid, from Chapter 5, into your marketing calendar. It becomes a mini-New Patient Machine, as you can track how each of your five approaches works with each of your five types of ideal patients, and you'll be gathering lots of useful data to analyze what marketing efforts are working best, not only in raw volume, but also in the number of ideal patients.

It should be obvious that if any doctor were to use all the techniques presented in this book it would generate hundreds of new patients every month. Very few doctors need that kind of new patient flow, and if you do, you may want to use some more advanced new patient attraction techniques, like radio and TV shows, advanced Internet marketing, high-profile blogs, major promotions, and more we'll cover at a future date.

For now, use the New Patient Machine technology to structure a new patient strategy that is consistent with your current level of play and the right size growth steps for you to feel fulfilled without being overwhelmed. You have dozens of new patient generating activities you can use—asking for referrals, networking with professionals, presenting talks, sponsoring promotions, using the Internet, putting back end items up front, and hundreds of permutations and combinations you can custom tailor to your particular liking.

By applying the science, philosophy, and art of the New Patients Every Day systems, you can always know where your attention is needed—do you need to build capacity, or do you have sufficient capacity, and you need to build attraction?

Are you gaining rapport in the new patient scenario, and are you asking questions to elicit values you can support with your communication?

Are you using a structured new patient approach, designed scientifically around your analysis of the data you've collected from your previous efforts?

Do you have a clear vision of ideal patients and your ideal practice, and the way you need to show up to create such a practice?

Do you have five-by-five grid and marketing calendar to guide your focus daily, weekly, monthly, and more, to help you hold yourself accountable?

Do you have an effective blend of hunting and farming, based on how hungry you are?

Remember, when you walk down the street, 90% of the people you see are not under chiropractic care, and 99% are not under your care. There are more than enough people to fill your practice with more ideal patients than you could possibly handle—new patients every day. It's the magnitude of your capacity and attraction that determines how many new patients you get, and how many visits you see.

Work on yourself, work on your practice, and work on bringing in new patients every day. Imagine if every chiropractor started just one new patient every day, what would happen?

Figure 50,000 chiropractors, attracting four new patients per week, or 200 per year. That would be 10,000,000 new chiropractic patients each year, meaning that we would hit critical mass (11% or so) in the fourth year. But since there will be some chiropractors who will not perform at that level, you, dear Doctor, may choose to bring in two, or three, or more new patients every day.

If you follow the rules of capacity and attraction, there's no limit to how many people you can help. The only boundaries are your imagination and your willingness to do what it takes. Please, help as many people as possible.

Points to Remember

1. The New Patient Machine has four gears—targeting ideal patients, building new patient capacity, setting effective new patient goals, and developing a marketing calendar that self-corrects and brings in new patients every day.

2. Target ideal patients with five steps—identify, locate, increase visibility, close effectively, and serve congruently.

3. Build capacity by understanding how you apply your time, energy, and resources.

4. Set goals that are both motivating and believable.

5. Compose a marketing calendar that will attract new patients at your desired rate.

Actions to Take

1. Using the "Right New Patient Flow For You" exercise, determine if you have sufficient capacity to handle the number of new patients you desire.

2. Using the 10%/20% rule, plot your course from where you are to where you want to be in practice volume and new patients.

3. Choose marketing events that will attract the kind of people you want, and insert those events into your marketing calendar so you have a specific game plan every single month without deviation.

Questions to Ponder

1. What qualities would you need to develop in yourself to hold yourself to these standards?

2. What would happen in your practice and your life if you executed on these opportunities?

3. Assuming that there are more than enough new patients to go around, how can you share these ideas with other chiropractors to add energy to making this world a better place?

This completes Chapter 8, The New Patient Machine, and brings this book to a close. I hope you enjoyed our work together, and that you will use these ideas to serve as many people as you can reach to make this world a healthier place, and to bring in New Patients Every Day.

Thank you for caring, and for loving what I love—I wish you abundance, success, and fulfillment in your practice and your life.

CLOSING REMARKS

You now have a series of systems that can be adapted to bring in the right number of the right kind of new patients for you. You have learned the philosophy of practice growth, growing capacity and filling it with attraction. You've learned that to create the best being and doing, you need to perform habits of excellence with optimal attitude and energy.

You've learned about the Practice Fulfillment Quotient, the five areas of your practice that help you troubleshoot where your attention is best invested to create your best practice—your identity, your practice philosophy, your new patient flow, your patient compliance, and your money management, which fit together to generate what you find fulfilling in practice.

So, you see now that attracting new patients every day doesn't happen in a vacuum—it's part of a system that is composed of smaller systems, and by wrapping your mind around this idea, you can break through and crack the code to attract all the new patients you want. I have coached many doctors who attracted fifty, sixty, seven, eighty new patients each month—one immensely talented doctor has attracted over 300 new patients in a calendar month, and often attracts 200 or more—but I never did that, and chances are you don't want to do it, either.

The beauty of the New Patients Every Day Systems™ is that they can be adjusted to any level of attraction, based on where you direct your attention. For some doctors, one new patient a day is about right—for some, too much, and for others, not nearly enough.

But new patients every day is just a metaphor—you can set the NPED dial to wherever you want it, and by adjusting the gears of the new patient machine—by targeting your ideal patients, by refining your procedures so you use your time effectively, by setting meaningful goals and developing a marketing calendar that has been scientifically proven to produce at the rate you desire—well, from there on it's a joyful ride, helping people, making money, and feeling fulfilled in your practice.

We explored six different categories of new patient strategies—referrals, networking with professionals, public speaking, promotions, Internet marketing, and back-end fronting. A systematic approach to any one of these categories could attract all the new patients you could handle.

You decide what type of artistry you want to apply. If you like to mix it up and keep it interesting, use the five-by-five marketing approach to keep lots of different marketing strategies in play, and change it up as often as you like. If you'd rather choose a method and master it, concentrate on just one or a few of these strategies and focus your resources there, again, until you wish to change it.

It's the movement of the four gears of the new patient machine that will determine how automatic your new patient attraction will become. Target your ideal patients—identify who you want, find them, get their attention, enroll them, and serve them well. Create the right new patient flow for you by analyzing your time capacity and calculating how to make your procedures as efficient as possible, and set goals that are both believable and motivating to keep them at the right level to preserve your momentum. Finally, insert your relevant marketing strategies into a marketing calendar, integrating your choice of techniques, using the six categories of new patient strategies as an artist's palette from which you can select or mix your colors.

If you want more children in the practice, increase your intention and adjust your strategy accordingly. If you learn a new technique that helps certain types of patients, develop a process to attract more of those. This system is infinitely flexible, and scalable to almost any volume.

This book is organized so you can use it as a reference, either to check in on specific new patient attraction techniques, or to explore newer, more expanded systems to build your new patient machine to work the way you want, to attract more new patients or a different blend.

That's the beauty of bringing in New Patients Every Day, or at whatever rate you prefer—when you understand the system, you can set it to any level of attraction, for any type of new patient, and you can change it any time you desire.

When you re-read this book, notice which of the tools you have already implemented, and which ones appealed to you but have not yet been applied. When is the right time to get those efforts in gear?

It will come back to you many times over to stay engaged with this material. If we share a dream of getting the chiropractic message to everyone so they can make an informed decision, then you can see why attracting more new patients gets us closer to that critical mass.

Our culture is suffering from a pandemic of brain stress the likes of which has never been seen or experienced. Between physical stress, mental stress, chemical stress, and electromagnetic stress, we have to withstand an onslaught of stressful forces every day. Chiropractic care can help get people back on track—and it's up to us to lead all those who will listen back to wellness and a better quality of life. No one is better equipped to do this than we are.

Chiropractic care can revolutionize the health and the lives of the people in our communities and beyond. Reach out and serve as many patients as possible, and let's pull together to make our world a healthier place. You'll help more people, make more money, and become a thought leader in your sphere of influence. And it can all move quickly in that direction when you bring in New Patients Every Day.

ACKNOWLEDGMENTS

This book was the culmination of thousands of hours of discussion with chiropractors about how they attract and process new patients. Therefore, my first acknowledgment goes to the chiropractic profession, as each doctor of chiropractic is charged with the responsibility of representing the entire profession with every new patient opportunity—hats off to all who enter the fray with the intention of helping people and making the world a healthier place.

There are many chiropractic mentors who have supported me in this endeavor. My partner at The Masters Circle, Dr. Bob Hoffman, generously shared his materials with me, without which this book would not be complete. Dr. Larry Markson first exposed me to the principles of success in chiropractic practice. Dr. Guy Riekeman inspired me from the time I was a student at NYCC to bring in patients for the right reason. Dr. Richard Van Rumpt and Dr. M. L. Rees served as technique giants who moved me to relentlessly pursue and conquer subluxation.

My primary communications teacher was Anthony Robbins, whose studies in human behavior revolutionized my practice and my life. Dr. Bob Bays introduced me to the enneagram, which became a vital filter through which I observed the new patient attraction process. I thank my key coaches at TMC, Alan Rousso, Brett Axelrod, Janice Hughes, Robert Kleinwaks, Barry Warren, Ken Freedman and Lisa Zinberg, and many others who helped me to formulate and refine these ideas on practice building and new patient generation.

Nothing I've done would have been possible without my wonderful family—my lovely wife, Regina, always the light of my life; my outstanding sons, Jeremy, Sean, and Dr. Daniel, at the time of publication just entering our glorious profession after completing his studies at Life West; and my late parents, Dr. Bill and Eileen Perman, may they rest in peace, who tirelessly served chiropractic in dozens of profound and meaningful ways. I love all of you more than I can say.

I appreciate my literary team—my coaches at Quantum Leap, including Steve Harrison, Geoffrey Berwind, Martha Bullen, and Brian Edmondson; firstediting.com, bookbaby.com, createspace.com, and Deana Riddle— you have all helped me become a better and more productive writer.

And finally, I acknowledge the chiropractic patient, the beneficiary of our hard work, who makes our dream of a healthier world real by engaging our services. Without the patient, we have no purpose—but with the patient, we can forge a new reality where nature prevails, the body is allowed to heal itself, and disease care gives way to health and wellness care for the betterment of our society. This dream is manifesting as we speak—and is a compelling reason to apply what you have learned here, for your pleasure and your patient's well-being.

RESOURCES

Thanks to:

The Masters Circle (Dr. Bob Hoffman 800-451-4514) www.themasterscircle.net
Free content: download free TMC App, download free TMC podcasts
Products: Masters Guide, Mastering The Message, The Edge Of Prosperity,
Identity Of A Healer, Tools Of Mastery, New Patients Every Day Boot
Camp, The Enneagram, Serum Thiol Testing

Drs. Patrick and Cynthia Porter, PorterVision.com, MindFit
Dr. Richard Barwell, NeuroInfiniti.com
Bob Mangat and Roger Lessard, website and Internet marketing, invigo.ca
Dr. Ed Osburn, Podcast Training, dred@thechiropracticphilanthropist.com
Brian Edmondson, Internetincomecoach.com
Kent Greenawalt, FootLevelers.com, Foundation For Chiropractic
Progress, F4CP.com
Dr. Ken and Lisa Davis, Natural Force healing, davisahs.com
Dr. Bill Doreste, CRT, cranialrelease.com
Dr. Mitch Mally, Extremity Adjusting, mrmally@live.com

Dr. Tedd Koren, KST, TeddKorenSeminars.com

Contact Reflex Analysis, CRAwellness.com, vervita.com

Dr. Brian Wolfs, Food Allergy Testing, hemocode.com

Chiropractic Leadership Alliance, Insight, subluxation.com

Dr. Clay Campbell, Dr. David Walls-Kaufman, serum thiol testing, contact TMC

Dr. Don Hayes, Alkalinity, GreensFirst.com

Neurological Relief Centers, nrc.md

Dr. Anna Saylor, vaneverychiropractic.com

Dr. Michael Leahy, ART activerelease.com

Dr. Ted Carrick, carrickbraincenters.com

International Systemic Health Organization, Harmonics

Special thanks to:

Jack Canfield

Dr. Robert Cialdini

Dr. Gerry Clum

Ryan Diess, *The Invisible Selling Machine*

Dvprompter.com

Dr. Patrick Gentempo

Dr. Jerry Greenberg

Dr. Christopher Kent

Dr. Brad Miller

Jeremy Perman

Dr. Karsten Petersen

Reputation.com

Tony Robbins

Sarah Santacroce, simplyadmins.ch

Dr. Scott Surasky

John Tabitha

In Memoriam

Stephen Covey

Dr. Major DeJarnette

Dr. Joe Flesia

Dr. Granville Frisbie

Dr. George Goodheart

Dr. M. T. Morter

Dr. Ron Pero

Dr. Vern Pierce

Dr. Glenn Stillwagon

Dr. Richard Van Rumpt

Dr. Dick Versendaal

Dr. Lowell Ward

Dr. Thomas LeRoy Whitehorne

ABOUT THE AUTHOR

Dennis Perman, DC, author, speaker, healer, and coach, has trained thousands of doctors of chiropractic and other wellness professionals and paraprofessionals for twenty-seven years. As co-founder of The Masters Circle, he has delivered hundreds of presentations to enthusiastic audiences throughout the US and Europe.

His innovative Capacity Technology™ provides a roadmap to practice success and personal growth. The co-author of The Masters Guide (with Drs. Bob Hoffman and Larry Markson), Dr. Perman has also written, produced, and recorded over sixty hours of original material on practice building, new patient attraction, communication, team building, personality engineering, self-development, and much more.

The executive producer of TMCtv, the world's largest online video success library for chiropractors, with over 350 hours of programming, Dennis also co-produced *MasterTalk* with Dr. Bob Hoffman and Jeremy Perman for fourteen seasons, 168 editions. He has published his *Message Of The*

Week eNewsletter every Monday for eighteen years, since September 1997, over 900 consecutive weeks, almost half a million words.

A pioneer in brain based wellness, with Drs. Hoffman, Barwell, Porter, Porter, Doreste, and other significant contributors too numerous to mention, Dennis helps chiropractors learn how to communicate their message from the inside out.

With "New Patients Every Day," he fills a long-time need—a reference book that teaches doctors of chiropractic how to get new patients.

"The tools and techniques in this book will evolve with new technology, but the systems are timeless and boundless—please use them to help as many people as you can."